Biochemistry of Body Weight Management

by
ASTHA DWIVEDI

Acknowledgements

First and foremost, I would like to thank God, the Almighty for having made everything possible and giving me the strength and courage to do this work. I acknowledge with gratitude my Supervisor **Prof. Abhay Kumar Pandey** and my Ex. Supervisor **Prof. Poonam Chandra Mittal** for their constant support, encouragement, immensely valuable ideas and suggestions and for going through the manuscript critically without which it was not possible to complete this work. I thank them for all the faith and belief they bestowed in me from the initial phase of the work. My association with them has also taught me to appreciate the value of persistent tolerance in the development of healthy scientific environment.

I would like to express my sincere thanks to, Prof. Shekhar Srivastava, Head of Department Biochemistry, for providing me his valuable suggestions and the necessary departmental research infrastructures. I am also thankful to Prof D. K. Gupta, Prof. Bechan Sharma, Prof S.I. Rizvi, Dr. Munish Kumar, Dr. Jalaj K Gour and Dr. Ujla Minhas.

I would like to owe my thanks to staff members of Department of Biochemistry for supporting me throughout my journey. I am grateful to all those volunteers who provided their blood samples without which it would have been impossible to do this work.

I heartily acknowledge the stimulating companionship and full cooperation of my friends Dr. Sharmistha Singh, Sandeep Kumar, Mr. Ramesh Kumar and Dr. Ashutosh Gupta. They helped me always when I needed their support and encouragement. We shared a lot of good moments in the lab and will always cherish as golden memories of my life.

I feel extremely proud and honoured to express my deepest sense of gratitude to my parents for their unconditional support, care and everlasting blessings. I also thank the contribution of all my family members for their affection, care and support.

I gratefully acknowledge the financial assistance by CSIR for CSIR-JRF NET and SRF fellowships and UGC for CRET fellowship. The DST- FIST and UGC-SAP facilities of Biochemistry Department are also acknowledged.

Astha Dwivedi

List of Abbreviations

%	- Percentage
ACD	- Acid Citrate Dextrose
CRP- C	- Reactive Protein
CuZn SOD	- Copper zinc Superoxide dismutase
CVD	- Cardiovascular disease
dl	- deciliter
EDTA	- Ethylene diamine tetraacetic acid
FBG	- Fasting Blood Glucose
FLOP	- Fluorescent Oxidation Product
FRAP	- Ferric Reducing Ability of Plasma
FRs	- Free Radicals
g/dl	- gram/deciliter
GAA	- Glacial Acetic Acid
GPx	- Glutathione peroxidase
GSH	- Reduced glutathione
GSSG	- Oxidized glutathione
H_2O_2	- Hydrogen peroxide
H_2O_2	- Hydrogen Peroxide
Hb	- Hemoglobin
HCl	- Hydrochloric acid
HDL-C	- High density lipoprotein
HO_2	- Hydroperoxyl radicals
IL-6	- Interleukin -6
LDL	- Low density Lipoprotein
LPO	- Lipid peroxidation
MDA	- Malondialdehyde
mM	- Millimolar
NHANES	- National Health and Nutrition Examination Survey
nmols/g	- Nano moles/gram
O_2	- Superoxide radical

O2	- Superoxide Anion
OH•-	- Hydroxyl Radical
OS	- Oxidative Stress
PBS	- Phosphate Buffered Saline
PRBCs	- packed Red Blood Cells
RBC	- Red Blood Cells
RNS	- Reactive Nitrogen Species
ROOH•	- Organic peroxide
ROS	- Reactive Oxygen Species
ROS	- Reactive Oxygen Species
SBP	- Systolic Blood Pressure
SOD	- Superoxide dismutase
T2DM	- Type 2 Diabetes Mellitus
TBA	- Thiobarbituric acid
TCA	- Trichloro acetic acid
TG	- Triglycerides
TNF-α	- Tumor necrosis factor
VLDL	- Very low density lipoprotein
WC	- Waist Circumference
Zn	- Zinc
μl	- Microlitre

Contents

INTRODUCTION 1
REVIEW OF LITERATURE 9
   2.1 Body weight Management: 9
   2.2 Definition of adult Overweight and Obesity: 10
      2.2.1. General Obesity: 10
      2.2.2. Central Obesity: 12
      2.2.3. Metabolically Healthy Obesity (MHO): 13
   2.4. Adipose Tissue and Obesity: 13
   2.5. Effect of age and gender on prevalence of Obesity: 16
      2.5.1. Age: 16
      2.5.2. Gender: 18
   2.6. Pathophysiology associated with obesity: 19
      2.6.1. Diabetes: 20
      2.6.2. Dyslipidaemia: 20
      2.6.3. Hypertension: 21
      2.6.4. Metabolic Syndrome: 21
   2.7. Role of Oxidative stress in obesity related diseases: 23
   2.8. Obesity and antioxidant capacity: 24
   2.9. Oxidative stress and mechanisms of cellular damage: role of free radicals ..25
      2.9.1. Oxidative damage to lipids: 26
      2.9.2. Oxidative damage to Proteins: 28
   2.10. Antioxidant defence mechanisms in the cells: 29
      2.10.1. Superoxide dismutase (CuZn SOD) 30
      2.10.2. Catalase: 30
      2.10.3. Glutathione peroxidase (GPx): 31
      2.10.4. Non-enzymatic defence: 32
      2.10.5. FRAP Assay: 32
   2.11. Obesity and inflammation: 33
      2.11.1. Tumor Necrosis Factor- alpha (TNF- α) and Obesity: 33
      2.11.2. Interleukin 6 (IL 6) and Obesity: 34
      2.11.3. C reactive protein (CRP) and Obesity: 34
METHODS AND MATERIALS **38**

3.1. Selection criteria for detection of metabolically healthy obesity (MHO): 38
3.2. Selection of Respondents: 38
3.3. Inclusion Criteria: 39
3.4. Exclusion criteria: 39
3.5. Study Design: 39
3.6. Further assessment of the individuals who fulfilled inclusion and exclusion criteria: 40
    3.6.1   Measurement of Body Mass Index and waist circumference: 40
    3.6.2   Division of respondents into Study groups: 40
3.7. Blood Collection, Processing and Storage: 42
3.8. Preparation of erythrocyte lysate: 43
3.9. Estimation of Haemoglobin (Hb): 43
3.10. Fasting Blood Glucose and Lipid profile: 43
3. 11 Assessment of Oxidative Stress Markers 44
    3.11.1 Hydroxyl radicals ($^\cdot$OH): 44
    3.11.2 Fluorescent Oxidation Products (FLOPs): 45
    3.11.3 Malondialdehyde (MDA): 45
    3.11.4 Protein Carbonyl (PCO): 45
3.12 Assessment of Antioxidant enzymes: 46
    3.12.1 Superoxide Dismutase activity (CuZn-SOD): 46
    3.12.2 Catalase (CAT): 46
    3.12.3 Glutathione Peroxidase (GPx) activity: 46
3.13. Total Antioxidant Activity (TAC) indexed as FRAP: 47
3.14. Measurement of Inflammatory Markers: 47
    3.14.1. Interleukin 6 (IL-6): 47
    3.14.2. Tumor Necrosis Factor alpha (TNF-α): 48
    3.14.3. C- Reactive Protein (CRP): 49
3.15. Statistical Analysis: 50
RESULTS AND DISCUSSION 51
SUMMARY AND CONCLUSION 141
REFERENCES 150
ANNEXURE 165

List of Tabel

Table 2.1.	WHO prescribed criteria to define obesity into different grades.	11
Table 4.1.1:	General characteristics of metabolically healthy non obese control (MHNO), metabolically healthy overweight (MHOw) and metabolically healthy obese (MHO).	51
Table 4.1.2:	NCEP ATP III diagnostic criteria for Met S and other clinical biochemical measures, to describe MHNO, MHOw and MHO phenotypes.	52
Table 4.1.3:	Results from Tukey's test for all parameters to assess pairwise significance between groups of metabolically healthy phenotypes.	53
Table 4.1.4.	Erythrocytic/plasma oxidative stress, antioxidant and inflammatory markers in MHNO, MHOW and MHO respondents.	55
Table 4.1.5:	Post Hoc analysis using Tukeys test to assess comparisons between groups.	56
Table 4.1.6:	Pearson's correlation coefficients to assess relationships of BMI with OS, antioxidant markers and inflammatory for MHNO, MHO_W and MHO.	59
Table 4.1.B1:	NCEP ATP III diagnostic criteria for MetS, other biochemical measures, OS markers and inflammatory markers defined by WHO and revised consensus guidelines for India.	66
Table 4.1.B2:	Post Hoc analysis using Tukeys' test to assess comparisons between groups.	68
Table 4.2.1	General characteristics of the three age groups (20-39, 40-59 and ≥60) in metabolically healthy Control (MHNO), MH overweight (MHOw) and Obese (MHO) respondents.	75
Table 4.2.2.	Age- wise distribution of Met S risk factors and other biochemical measures in MHNO, MHOw and MHO group respondents.	77
Table 4.2.3.	Age- wise distribution of erythrocytic and plasma oxidative stress markers and antioxidant status of MHNO, MHOw and MHO respondents.	80
Table 4.2.4.	Age- wise distribution of inflammatory markers in groups of MHNO, MHOw and MHO.	83
Table 4.2.4.	Impact of Age on Body Mass Index, and Oxidative stress (OS) indicators in MHNO, MHOw and MHO respondents.	88
Table 4.3.1.	General characteristics of Male and Female respondents assigned to MHNO, MHOw and MHO.	99

Table 4.3.2.	Gender wise comparison of risk factors of MetS in metabolically healthy non obese controls (MHNO), MH overweight (MHOw) and MH obese (MHO) respondents.	100
Table 4.3.3.	Gender wise comparisons between males and females of MHNO, MHOw and MHO groups with regard to marker of Erythrocytic and plasma oxidative stress markers, antioxidants and redox status.	103
Table 4.3.4:	Gender wise comparisons between male and female of MHNO, MHOw and MHO group with regard to inflammatory markers	106
Table 4.3.4.	Interrelationships between oxidative stress (OS) markers, body weight and body mass index (BMI), in male and female respondents of MHNO, MHOw and MHO.	108
Table 4.4.1:	General characteristics of MHNO and respondents suffering from metabolically healthy General Obesity (MHGO) and Central Obesity(MHCO) groups.	114
Table 4.4.2:	NCEP ATP III prescribed diagnostic measures and other clinical biochemical measures of MHNO, General obesity (MHGO) and Central obesity (MHCO) groups.	115
Table 4.4.3:	Plasma and Erythrocytic oxidative stress markers, and circulating inflammatory markers in respondents of metabolically healthy non obese (MHNO), MHGO and MHCO groups.	117
Table 4.4.4:	Interrelationships among oxidative stress (OS), antioxidants and inflammatory markers with body mass index (BMI) and waist circumference (WC), as indicated by Pearson's correlation coefficients r.	121
Table 4.5.1:	General characteristics of respondents assigned to metabolically healthy obese (MHO) and metabolically unhealthy obese (MUHO) groups	130
Table 4.5.2:	NCEP ATP III prescribed diagnostic measures and other clinical biochemical measures of respondents assigned to metabolically healthy obese (MHO) and metabolically unhealthy obesity (MUHO)	130
Table 4.5.3:	Erythrocytic and plasma oxidative stress markers of metabolically healthy obese (MHO) and metabolically unhealthy obesity (MUHO).	132
Table 4.5.4:	Interrelationships between oxidative stress (OS) markers with waist circumference (WC), as indicated by Pearson's correlation coefficients r.	134
Table 4.5.5:	AUC of OS indices for predicting their use in distinguishing metabolically unhealthy obesity with metabolic syndrome (MUHO) and metabolically healthy obesity (MHO).	136

List of Figures

Figure 2.1. White adipose tissue expansion in obesity. 15

Figure 2.2. Pathophysiological Mechanism in metabolically unhealthy obesity (MUHO) with Metabolic Syndrome 22

Figure 2.3: Interrelationship between obesity and oxidative stress 24

Figure 2.4: Mechanism of Oxidative Stress in cellular damage 29

Figure 3.1. Flowchart for the selection and distribution of respondents for Chapters 1-3. 42

Figure 3.2. Flowchart for processing of blood and fractions used for biochemical estimations. 44

Figure 3.3. Standard Curve for IL-6 48

Figure 3.4. Standard Curve for TNF –α. 49

Figure 4.1.1: Relative per cent difference of NCEP ATP III diagnostic criteria for Met S, and related biochemical parameters between MHNO and MHOw, MHNO and MHO, and MHOw and MHO. 54

Figure 4.1.2: Relative per cent difference of biochemical parameters between MHNO and MHOw, MHNO and MHO and MHOw and MHO, with regard to (a) serum hydroxyl radicals (•OH), plasma fluorescent oxidation products (FLOP), malondialdehyde (MDA) and protein carbonyl (PCO), (b) CuZn Superoxide dismutase (CuZn SOD), glutathione peroxidase (GPx), catalase (CAT) and ferric reducing ability of plasma (FRAP), and (c) C reactive protein (CRP), tumor necrosis factor alpha (TNF –α), interleukin 6 (IL- 6). 58

Fig 4.1.3 (a) OH Rad vs BMI (b). FLOP vs BMI 65

Figure 4.2.1 (a) Age vs body weight   Figure 4.2.1(b) Age vs BMI 76

Fig 4.2.1. Relationship between age and (a) body weight (b) BMI in MHNO, MHOw and MHO respondents. 76

Figure. 4.2.1: Age- wise distribution of (a) OH Radicals, (b) FLOP, (c) MDA, (d) PCO, (e) erythrocytic SOD, (f) erythrocytic CAT, (g) plasma GPx, (h) FRAP, (i) CRP, (j) TNF alpha, (k) IL 6 in MHNO, MHOw and MHO respondents. 87

Figure 4.4.1: Relative per cent difference of biochemical parameters between MHNO and MHGO, MHNO and MHCO, and MHCO and MHGO, with regard to (a) serum hydroxyl radicals (•OH), plasma fluorescent oxidation products (FLOP), malondialdehyde (MDA) and protein carbonyl (PCO), (b) CuZn Superoxide dismutase (CuZn SOD), glutathione peroxidase (GPx), catalase (CAT) and ferric reducing ability of plasma

	(FRAP), and (c) C reactive protein (CRP), tumor necrosis factor alpha (TNF –α), interleukin 6 (IL- 6)..120
Figure 4.4.2:	Correlation graphs for (a) OH Rad vs WC (b) FLOP vs WC (c) MDA vs WC, (d) PCO vs WC, (e) CuZn SOD vs WC, (f) CAT vs WC, (g) GPx vs WC, (h) FRAP vs WC, (i) CRP vs WC, (j) TNF alpha vs WC (k) IL 6 vs WC among MHNO, MHGO and MHCO respondents. 124
Figure 4.5.1:	Relative per cent difference of NCEP ATP III diagnostic criteria for Met S, and related biochemical parameters between MHO and MUHO group..131
Figure 4.5.2:	Relative per cent difference in oxidative stress markers between MHO and MUHO experimental groups. 133
Figure: 4.5.3	Relative per cent difference in inflammatory markers CRP, TNF alpha and IL 6 MHO and MUHO. 133
Figure 4.5.4	Area under receiver operating characteristic curve (AUC) for oxidative stress markers (a) MDA, (b) PCO, (c), CuZn SOD, (d) CAT, (e) GPx and (f) FRAP. 135

Chapter-1

INTRODUCTION

The importance of maintenance of body weight in humans throughout adult life to promote good health is being increasingly recognized. While body weight can be both lower and higher than normal, overweight has attracted more attention, and is considered to be one of the most challenging health risks of present time. The last few decades have seen a rapid rise in research linking increase in body weight to several adverse effects on health due to predisposition to many diseases such as diabetes, hypertension, chronic heart diseases, osteoarthritis, cancer, and consequent reduced life expectancy [WHO 2000, Weiss R, Dziura J, Burgert TS et al., 2004]. A common correlate of these conditions is the associated production of free radicals and consequent oxidative stress.

The most common causes of increased weight are decrease in energy requirements due to reduced physical activity and lowering of metabolic activity. In women, this has been linked to decrease in estrogen around menopause. Weight gain has also been observed in men but the issue of age related weight gain in relation to gender has not received as much attention.

Despite the unequivocal role of physical activity in maintenance of weight, recent researches indicate that a one-to-one relationship between energy intake and expenditure is not always found and the process of body weight management over a lifetime is very complex. Several issues have been found to be associated with excess body fat and encompass dietary history, quantity and quality of food intake, physical activity and exercise, psychological stresses, sleep patterns, environmental toxicity, exposure to tobacco, caffeine etc, as well as metabolic, endocrine and genetic issues. Living beings have evolved through food shortages, so they are genetically and metabolically predisposed to assimilate and store as much energy as possible in times of food surplus, and hold on to the stores by changing metabolism, even when energy intakes are lowered. This is a major reason which complicates body weight management.

Obesity is defined as metabolic condition of increased adipose tissue mass where excess nutrient intake increases the body weight as compared to energy usage [Gray DS., 1989]. Excessive accumulation of triacylglycerols (TAG, fat), may alter the free fatty acids metabolism and results in TAG storage in muscles, liver, visceral regions around the organs, waist, thighs that causes obesity. Obesity is considered as one of the most important risk factor in expansion and succession of insulin resistance, dyslipidemia, metabolic syndrome and cardiovascular diseases.

The Body mass index (BMI) is the most accepted obesity index marker according to World Health Organization (WHO), to define obesity into different grades, which is calculated by dividing the weight in kilograms by the square of the height in meters (m^2). WHO categorizes adult obesity into different grades, those with BMI$\leq$25 kg/m^2 as non-obese; 25-30 kg/m^2 as overweight, and BMI$\geq$30 kg/m^2 as obese [WHO, 1995]. Previous studies have shown that BMI is strongly associated with percent body fat in even in younger and middle aged individuals [Dietz WH, Robinson TN, 2005; NHLBI Expert Panel, 2002]. BMI is a good indicator of percent body fat but much controversy arises over the use of BMI because it does not discriminate between free fat mass and fatty mass hence the concept of waist circumference (WC) an index marker of central obesity, has been introduced by WHO to assess metabolic health issues associated with central obesity [WHO, 2008].

The etiology of excess body fat has been linked to number of risk factors independently or rather how they interact with one another. The major risk factor of obesity is energy imbalance between energy intake and storage. This energy imbalance is partially a result of modern lifestyles, urbanization, quantity and quality of food intake, genetic environmental factors [Malik, VS., Willett WC., Hu FB., 2013].

It has been well known that obesity is associated with number of metabolic complications like insulin resistance, diabetes mellitus, metabolic syndrome and cardiovascular diseases. However, not all obese people exhibit metabolic complications, representing a distinct subset of obese individuals without occurrence of metabolic complications known as metabolically healthy obesity (MHO). Till date there is no universally accepted classification for MHO, but NCEP ATP III criteria to define Met S is most acceptable in clinical practice. According to NCEP ATP III criteria MHO phenotypes may be defined as absence of metabolic syndrome risk factors. MHO phenotypes usually have normal lipid blood profile, fasting plasma glucose, less visceral adipose tissue and reduces inflammatory profile as compared to obese with metabolic syndrome [Häring SN, Hu HU, Schulze FB. et al., 2013]. The prevalence of metabolically healthy obese (MHO) phenotypes exhibit different degree of variability ranges between 10 to 34 %. The prevalence of MHO is more in younger and middle age people, but decreases as age advances in both gender and is more widespread in women than men [Van Vliet-Ostaptchouk JV, Nuotio ML, Slagter SN. et al., 2014].

Recent consensus report by Ahirwar [Ahirwar R and Mondal PR. et al., 2019] has reported that worldwide 1.9 billion adults are overweight and 650 million are obese and 2.8 million deaths are reported due to overweight or obesity. Its prevalence rate is rapidly increasing worldwide at all stages of life in both developed as well as in developing countries. As we age, there is progressive decrease in fat free body mass (FFM or skeletal muscle), while percent body fat reaches maximum levels at the age of 60 to 70. After the age of 70 FFM and body fat both tends to decrease, indicating the redistribution of subcutaneous or body fat is associated with aging [Gallagher D, Visser M, De Meersman RE et al., 1997]. Gender or sex is one of the essential factors that is affecting prevalence rate of obesity. Pattern of body fat distribution, adipose tissue storage and metabolism, represent gender disparities. Females have higher percentage of body fat and have less free fatty mass than males of same BMI group, indicating the biological differences among them [Power ML and Schulkin J., 2008]. In females, menopause affects body fat distribution that may increase the risk of weight gain (obesity) on health.

Another area of intense study with regard to the obesity and its relationship with chronic low grade systemic inflammation in adipose tissue, due to activation of the innate immune system that leads to development of oxidative stress and proinflammatory state. As a result, oxidative stress induced inflammatory markers has been hypothesized to be pathogenesis and progression of various obesity related metabolic complications like diabetes mellitus, metabolic syndrome, and cardiovascular diseases [Xu, H., Barnes, GT., Yang, Q. et al., 2003].

Oxidative stress is results of imbalance between prooxidant and antioxidant defence system that give rise to excess production of highly reactive free radical species, mainly reactive oxygen species (ROS) and reactive nitrogen species (RNS) [Roberts CK and Sindhu KK., 2009]. These species are highly reactive which makes them potentially very dangerous. Different radicals have very different chemical reactivity and mostly denoted by superscript dot. The structural and biochemical changes induced by reactive oxygen species are believed to be major cause of age related diseases including obesity. A most important hypothesis in this theory is that unpaired free radicals and their precursors may be produced endogenously (within the body) during normal catabolic/anabolic metabolic processes or exogenously (outside the body) from sources such as cigarette, smoking, pollutants. Free radical mediated attack on cell membranes and lipoproteins results in the lipid peroxidation measured in terms of malondialdehyde (MDA), attack on protein causes protein carbonylation (measured in terms of protein carbonyl, PCO) whereas attack on DNA results in the alterations in DNA bases implicated in cancer [Marrocco I, Altieri F, Peluso I et al., 2017]. Free radicals are made in the human body and antioxidants defence systems have evolved to protect against reactive free radicals. The redox homeostasis balance is maintained by various non enzymatic and enzymatic antioxidants known as superoxide dismutase (SOD), catalase (CAT), and glutathione peroxidase (GPx). This is accomplished by a set of antioxidant enzymes namely, superoxide dismutase (SOD), catalase (CAT), and glutathione peroxidase (GPx).

These enzymes are present as metallozymes. SOD is a metalloprotein present as CuZn SOD, found in cytosol and mitochondria, which catalyze the conversion of superoxide to hydrogen peroxide. The hydrogen peroxide generated by SOD is mostly removed by the GPx. Catalase are metallozymes that convert the hydrogen peroxide to water and oxygen, in presence of either iron or manganese cofactor. This protein is mostly present in peroxisomes of eukaryotic cells. Previous studies reported that the level of antioxidant enzymes have been found to decrease in obese subjects as compared to controls, leading to alterations in redox balance and total antioxidant capacity.[Venturini D, Simão AN, Scripes NA et al. 2012].

Previous studies reported that obesity is characterized by chronic low grade inflammation, which can lead to development of oxidative stress, the ultimate cause of obesity complications [Furukawa S, Fujita T, Shimabukuro M et al., 2004]. Inflammation is ordered sequence of physiological response of the organisms to maintain organ/tissue homeostasis. Obesity is medical condition of excess adipose tissue storage in form of triacylglycerides (TAG) [Karalis KP, Giannogonas P, Kodela E et al. 2009]. Excess storage of TAG in adipose tissue causes activation of proinflammatory adipocytokines and other inflammatory markers [Karalis KP, Giannogonas P, Kodela E et al. 2009]. In this context, tumor necrosis factor alpha (TNF alpha) plays a significant role in pathogenesis of obesity related comorbidities. Later, elevated level of circulating TNF alpha induces secretion of other proinflammatory cytokine IL-6, adiponectin, monocyte chemo attractant protein-1 (MCP-1), and CRP which directly play an important role in progression of insulin resistances, abdominal obesity and later T2DM and CVD. [Shoelson SE, Lee J, Goldfine Ab et al., 2006].

The erythrocytes are an early model for studies of oxidative stress. They are small, enucleated and biconcave, lacking cell organelles such as endoplasmic reticulum and mitochondria. Hence, their oxygen consumption is very low. Apart from their primary role in transporting oxygen to tissue and carbon dioxide to lungs, they are found to contain numerous complex enzymes some of them are necessary for their own metabolic need. They are the target for oxidative reaction because of their relatively high molecular oxygen tension and presence of haemoglobin and a plasma membrane rich in polyunsaturated fatty acids (PUFA). The erythrocytes are the most highly adapted cells in the body. They have an effective antioxidant mechanism to prevent and neutralize OS induced damage. Hence, it was decided to include parameters of OS and inflammation as studies on the biochemistry of body weight management.

Various models of research are used to answer questions related to human health and diseases. Animal models have been used because they allow data collection in controlled conditions, with minimization of inter individual variations. They have been popular, but subtle and obvious differences between humans and rat models (animals) in terms of anatomy, physiology and cellular metabolism make it complicated to apply research data derived from rat and other animal studies to human conditions, and accurately translating information from rat studies can be an exercise making an assumption.

A research group from the Vanderbilt University Medical Centre describe some of the trouble in animal models in their 2004 research article: The design of animal "studies"; The particular disease studied from animals are not truly similar to human disease (developed in long time period) but are partial representation of them", and in most cases data derived from animal studies do not assess the genetic variation induced by nature and its effect on phenotypic expression automatically controls many independent and dependent variables that can confound human studies [Wisdom, SJ., Wilson, R., McKillop, JH., et al. 1991]. According to Hackam et al (2006), [Hackam DG. and Redelmeier DA., 2006] physicians and patient should remain careful about extrapolating the data and conclusions of prominent animal studies to the care of human disease, even high quality animal research will replicate poorly in human clinical trials. According to Food and Drug Administration, 2006, nine out of ten trial drugs fail in clinical phase studies because we cannot accurately predict the mode of action of these trail drugs in individuals based on experimental animal studies. Hence for successful biomedical experimentation of the diagnosis and treatment of human diseases, the current approach is based on multiple artificial conditions in animal models, should be replaced by more relevant alternatives and return to an emphasis on clinical research and public health attention to preventative measures.

Therefore for this study, the human model was selected for better understanding of a realistic in vivo model to assess the relationship among obesity induced OS and inflammatory markers. The present study was undertaken to study Indian MH adults aged 20 to 80 years to assess the impact of their BMI on selected biochemical markers. The study was conducted with five objectives as follows:

(1) To compare metabolically healthy (MH) non obese controls, overweight and obese respondents with regard to NCEP ATP III Met S risk factors, markers of oxidative stress, redox balance and inflammation.

349 Metabolically Healthy (MH) respondents were divided into three groups: 100 metabolically healthy non obese controls (MHNO), 147 overweight (MHOw) and 102 obese (MHO) respondents.

(2) To compare metabolically healthy (MH) non obese controls (MHNO), metabolically healthy overweight (MHOw) and metabolically healthy obese (MHO) respondents with regard to NCEP ATP III Met S risk factors, markers of oxidative stress, redox balance and inflammation in relation to age.

The study population aged 20-80 years was divided into three age groups, young adults group (YA, 20-39 years), middle aged adults group (MA, 30-59 years), and elderly age group (EA, >60 years).

(3) To assess gender-specific association of NCEP ATP III MetS risk factors, oxidative stress, redox balance and inflammatory markers in metabolically healthy(MH) non obese controls (MHNO), overweight (MHOw) and obese (MHO) respondents.

The metabolically healthy non obese control (MHNO) group comprised of 56 males and 44 females, MH overweight (MHOw) group comprised of 74 males and 73 females and the MH obese (MHO) group comprised of 60 males and 42 females.

(4) To compare metabolically healthy (MH) non obese controls (MHNO), and those with general obesity (MHGO) or central obesity (MHCO) with regard to

NCEP ATP III MetS risk factors, markers of oxidative stress, redox balance and inflammation.

Metabolically healthy (MH) respondents were divided into three groups: 100 MH non obese controls (MHNO), 71 MH respondents with general obesity (MHGO) and 77 MH respondents with central obesity (MHCO).

(5) To compare metabolically healthy obese (MHO) and metabolically unhealthy obese (MUO) with regard to NCEP ATP III Met S risk factors, markers of oxidative stress, redox balance and inflammation.

Respondents comprising of two groups: 102 metabolically healthy obese (MHO) and 102 metabolically unhealthy obese (MUO) respondents were compared.

Chapter-2

REVIEW OF LITERATURE

2.1 Body weight Management:

Maintenance of body weight is a complex phenomenon requiring intricate homeostatic control. It has been under active scientific investigation because of its importance for health. Control of body weight involves maintenance within a small range beyond which a person may be designated underweight or overweight. Both aberrations can be associated with unhealthy outcomes. There is no clear consensus framework of body weight homeostasis but there seems little doubt that overweight/obesity constitute a more harmful condition, and has therefore attracted more attention. It is considered to be one of the most challenging health risks of present time [WHO, 2000]. Hence, the present study is focused on biochemical correlates of various overweight and obesity conditions.

Though obesity and its related complications have been recognized for thousands of years by Hippocrates [Haslam D, 2007], the last few decades have seen a rapid rise in research linking increase in body weight to several adverse effects on health due to predisposition to many diseases such as diabetes, hypertension, chronic heart diseases, osteoarthritis, cancer, and consequent reduced life expectancy.

It is important to understand the etiological factors that contribute to obesity. Obesity results due to an imbalance between energy intake and requirement. The most common cause of overweight and obesity is decrease in energy requirements due to reduced physical activity, and lowering of metabolic activity. Despite the unequivocal role of physical activity in maintenance of weight, recent researches indicate that a one-to-one relationship between energy intake and expenditure is not always found and the process of body weight management over a lifetime is very complex. Several issues have been found to be connected with excess body fat, and encompass dietary history, quantity and quality of food intake, physical activity and exercise, psychological stresses, sleep patterns, environmental toxicity, exposure to tobacco, caffeine etc, as well as metabolic, endocrine and genetic issues. History has witnessed longer periods of food shortage than excess, due to famines and floods. Metabolism has therefore evolved to hold on to available nutrients, by modifying metabolism, even when energy intakes are lowered. On the other hand, excess availability of food is a recent evolutionary phenomenon, and the human body is not metabolically evolved to adjust to it. This is a major reason which complicates management of body weight.

Obesity is characterized by excess body fat accumulation in adipose tissues that is reported to negatively affect metabolic health. The extent of comorbidities have been found to be linked to the quantity of adipose tissue but the distribution of this adipose tissue is also found to be very important. Another recent and interesting observation is that the adverse effects are not seen in all cases of obesity, and have been linked to specific genetics. These issues lead to understanding obesity in its various forms. The study of Central obesity, General obesity and a possible distinct phenotype designated as Metabolically Healthy Obesity. These categories of obesity currently occupy in depth and extensive scientific investigation, which are also the objective of the current research endeavour.

Hence, it is imperative to understand the various features associated with excess weight accumulation.

2.2 Definition of adult Overweight and Obesity:

2.2.1. General Obesity:

Obesity is commonly measured by Body Mass Index (BMI) as recommended by World Health Organization [WHO, 1995]. BMI is calculated by dividing body weight (Kg) by height squared (m^2). BMI is the most accepted obesity index which is used by all racial populations to identify the fraction of people with a high risk of an undesirable health state that warrants a public health or clinical intervention. WHO categorizes obesity in adults into different grades as described in Table 2.1.

Table 2.1. WHO prescribed criteria to define obesity into different grades.

	BMI Kg/m²	Obesity Class	Disease Risk* Relative to Normal Weight and Waist Circumference	
			Men≤102 cm(≤40 cm) Women≤88 cm(≤35 cm)	Men>102 cm(>40 cm) Women>102 cm(>40 cm)
Underweight	<18.5		-	-
Normal	18.5-24.9		-	-
Overweight	25-29.9		Increased	High
Obesity	30-34.9	I	High	Very High
	35-39.9	II	Very High	Very High
Extremely Obesity	≥40	III	Extremely High	Extremely High

Although the WHO advocated guidelines are still universally accepted, the last several years have witnessed a debate on requirement of ethnic-specific BMI cut-offs for different populations in the light of scientific evidence. According to some studies [Misra A, 2015], Asian populations have different associations between percentage of body fat, BMI, and metabolic health risks than do Caucasian populations. In 2004, a WHO Expert Consultative Committee [WHO Expert Consultation, 2004] addressed this debate and concluded that while the proportion of Asian people showing high risk of insulin resistance (IR) and cardiovascular disease (CVD) at lower BMI cut offs but available data do not necessarily indicate a clear BMI cut-off point for all Asian population for overweight or obesity. The BMI cut-off point for observed risk varies from 22 kg/m2 to 25 kg/m2 in different Asian populations; for high risk it varies from 26 kg/m2 to 31 kg/m2, so the committee did not recommend redefining cut-off points for each population separately, and agreed that the WHO BMI cut-off points should be retained as international classifications.

Although, BMI is the most acceptable index marker for categorizing metabolic health issues and is highly correlated with percent body fat but there are some limitations too. Thus, a high BMI is a measure of General Obesity. It does not distinguish between fat free mass (muscle mass) and fatty mass nor does it indicate anything about fat distribution. The metabolic health issues related to obesity depend on pattern of body fat distribution. For example, individual with high amount of subcutaneous fat (fat located beneath skin, hips and thighs) have fewer health risks than those with central obesity (visceral fat, fat around organs). There are many anthropometric indices to measure central obesity like waist circumference (WC), waist to hip ratio (WHR).

2.2.2. Central Obesity:

Central obesity is one of the most important risk factors for metabolic syndrome. WHO has recommended measurement of waist circumference (WC) combined with body mass index to assess metabolic health issues associated with obesity [WHO, 2008]. It is well accepted that centrally distributed fat is more pathogenic than subcutaneous fat, leading to various health consequences. Therefore, the Adult Treatment Panel III (ATP III) report of the National Cholesterol Education Program (NCEP) (NCEP ATP III) incorporated waist circumference as an individual risk factor for metabolic syndrome [Kelli H M, Corrigan F E, Heinl R E et al. 2017]. Excess visceral fat is associated with metabolic syndrome in both genders, and this extra visceral fat leads to adipocyte hypertrophy, macrophage infiltration, endothelial cell activation that leads to development of chronic low grade inflammation which is associated with increased oxidative stress, and over activity of nuclear factor kappa b pathway (NF-κB) [BondiaPons I, Ryan L, Martinez J A., 2012]. The NF-κB pathway up regulates the genes of pro inflammatory cytokines and chemokines such as TNF-α, IL-6, and IL-1, that leads to inflammatory state in adipose tissue causing various metabolic dysfunctions.

There is one more category of obesity which is a new area of study and has recently come in for widespread discussion as a distinct phenotype. This is known as Metabolically Healthy Obesity.

2.2.3. Metabolically Healthy Obesity (MHO):

Obesity is characterized by excess body fat and is associated with health consequences like type 2 diabetes mellitus dyslipidemia and metabolic syndrome. However, these cardiometabolic complications are not developed in all obese subjects and in 1985 Sims [Sims EAH., 1982] suggested the concept of metabolically healthy obesity [MHO]. MHO is a unique subset of obesity without any metabolic complications. Hence MHO individuals have lower proportion of visceral fat, normal blood pressure, favorable lipid profile, normal glucose metabolism and insulin sensitive despite having an excessive amount of body fat. [Pajunen P, Kotronen A, Korpi-Hyovalti E, et al., 2011; Karelis AD. and Rabasa-Lhoret R., 2008]. They are reported to have substantially lower risk of metabolic perturbations [Jung CH, Lee WJ, Song KH., 2017]. Currently, there are no universally accepted classification criteria to define individuals of MHO but the NCEP ATP III diagnostic criteria of metabolic syndrome is most acceptable in clinical practice to define MHO individuals on the basis of presence or absence of metabolic syndrome [NCEP, 2010; Karelis AD and Rabasa-Lhoret R.. 2008]. Metabolically healthy obesity is associated with normal metabolic regulation, which is largely dependent on normal adipose tissue function in response to excess nutrient supply. In normal situations, adipose tissue stores excess nutrient in the form of triglyceride synthesized from free fatty acids and in fasting states, triglycerides undergo lipolysis and release free fatty acids to provide energy. The whole process is regulated by secretion of adipokines and leptin. Metabolically healthy obese respondents have been reported to have lower oxidative stress induced inflammation and diminished adipose tissue macrophage infiltration in comparison to unhealthy obese individuals [Primeau V, Coderre L, Karelis AD et al., 2011]. Since obesity is a consequence of accumulated adipose tissue, it is important to understand the links between the two.

2.4. Adipose Tissue and Obesity:

Adipose tissue is a metabolically dynamic endocrine organ, playing a crucial role in regulation of energy storage. This regulation is achieved by storing energy as fat in the form of triglycerides (TGs) in periods of energy excess and releasing it in the form of fatty acids to provide energy requirements during fasting. Triglycerides which are stored in adipocytes, are first separated into their parts (three fatty acids and one glycerol molecule) in the presence of lipoprotein lipase (LPL), released from adipose tissues. Glycerol remains in the blood while free fatty acids are transported to adipocytes where they are again transformed into triglycerides and stored in lipid droplets. Adipose tissues are divided into two major categories: the brown adipose tissues (BAT) and the white adipose tissues (WAT). BAT is composed of multilocular adipocytes with abundant mitochondria that oxidize lipids to produce high amount of heat, through the action of uncoupling protein (UCP–1) found in the inner membrane of mitochondria which is responsible for thermogenic activity of tissue. BAT is mainly present in newborn of humans and in hibernating animals.

In contrast, white adipose tissue (WAT) is contains one single lipid droplet which is responsible for fat storage. WAT is heterogeneous in nature, with different major locations in the body, mainly subcutaneous adipose tissue (SAT) and visceral adipose tissue (VAT). Apart from adipocytes, it consists of wide variety of cells such as preadipocytes, fibroblasts, nerve cells, endothelial and vascular smooth muscle cells, immune cells (B and T cells), macrophages and neutrophils [Nishimura S, Manabe I, Nagasaki M. et al., 2009; Elgazar-Carmon V, Rudich A, Hadad N et al., 2008]. The fat depots of subcutaneous and visceral adipose tissue display distinct characteristics at the level of gene expression profile, as well as differences in regulation of whole body energy storage in the form of triglyceride storage and release [Tchkonia T, Thomou T, Zhu Y. et al., 2013].

In obesity, there is huge increase in white adipose tissues due to adipose tissue remodeling observed as changes in the size (hypertrophy) and number (hyperplasia) of the adipocytes. Such hypertrophic-hyperplastic remodeling governs the metabolic and cardiovascular outcome of associated diseases [Spiegelman BM and Flier JS., 1996]. Progenitor cells (pre adipocyte) have 80 % of subcutaneous adipose tissue and 20 % of visceral adipose tissue, which could explain that the expansion of visceral adipose tissue by hypertrophy predisposes to metabolic syndrome, diabetes, insulin resistance whereas, expansion of subcutaneous adipose tissue by hyperplasia represent the protective nature of these depots for lipid excess and thus protecting organs (liver, heart and muscles) from fatty infiltration. [McLaughlin T, Lamendola C, Liu A et al.,

2011]. Adipose tissue is metabolically dynamic organ and subject to a continuous process of hypertrophic – hyperplasic remodeling as per availability of energy intake which is important for maintaining tissue health. But under constant excess caloric intake condition this process is become unregulated, leading to death of adipocytes due to recruitment and activation of M1 macrophages, mast cells, dendritic cells and proinflammatory cytokines. [Lee MJ, Wu Y, Fried SK., 2010]. Activation of hypertrophic remodeling altered the level of proinflammatory cytokines. In parallel hyperplasic division of adipose tissue protect the obese individuals against adverse effects caused by lipotoxic systemic effect of excess free fatty acids. Thus, there is clear distinction between healthy and unhealthy expansion of adipose tissue. The unhealthy or pathological expansion of adipose tissue is linked with hypertrohic division, inducing M1 macrophages activation and infiltration, limited development of circulatory blood vessels, causing hypoxia, chronic oxidative stress and inflammatory state. The hyperplasic or healthy expansion of adipose tissue is associated with organized expansion of the fatty mass that leads to development of metabolically healthy obesity (MHO). Such individuals represent increased subcutaneous tissue with minimal induction of inflammation [Sun K, Kusminski CM, Scherer PE., 2011].

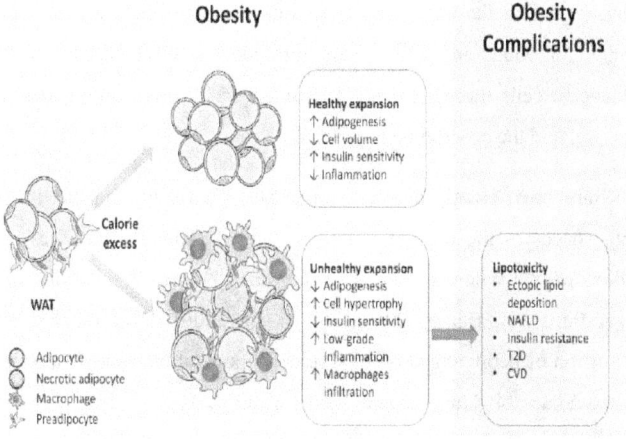

[Adopted from Longo M et al., 2019]

Figure 2.1. White adipose tissue expansion in obesity.

White adipose tissue responds to caloric excess through a healthy or unhealthy expansion. Healthy expansion through adipocyte hyperplasia protects against the metabolic complications of obesity. Unhealthy expansion through adipocyte hypertrophy promotes the obesity-associated metabolic complications. WAT, white adipose tissue; T2D, type 2 diabetes; NAFLD, non-alcoholic fatty liver disease; CVD, cardiovascular.

2.5. Effect of age and gender on prevalence of Obesity:

2.5.1. Age:

Aging is an inevitable phenomenon in all organisms. It refers to a multidimensional process of physical, psychological and social changes. Several theories have been put forward from time to time to explain the phenomenon of aging. Of these, one of the currently most accepted theories is the free radical theory [Harman D., 1992]. According to this, oxidative stress increases as a person ages, and may be the cause of a variety of age related diseases. Endogenous antioxidant systems and exogenous nutrients help in mitigating the harmful effects of oxidative stress. The last few years have brought many insights into the fundamental mechanisms of aging, showing that aging begins at the very early stages of life, and one's choices and the life styles throughout youth and adult years influence how one ages. The accumulation of damage to cells throughout life is influenced by a person's genes, food, amount of exercise, and the environment.

The number of elderly persons in the world is rising, and this is a consequence of rapid strides in the medical sciences. Global estimates indicate that there are 605 million people who are older than 65 years [World Population Ageing Highlights, 2019; Purty AJ, Bazroy J, Kar M. et al., 2006]. Over the last few decades, the proportion of people aged 60 plus (elderly population) is increased by 300 percent in United States of America and Asia [WHO., 2011; Thomas T, Ruth B, Konard J., 2001]. In some developed countries the number of older people will be twice the number of children. India is a developing country, where the proportion of young, middle and elderly age population are constantly increasing, whereas the age group of

0 to 14 years is decreasing. In 1991, the population of elderly age group was 6.7 % of total population, is expected to increase to more than 10 % by the year 2021 [Ministry of Statistics & Programme Implementation. Government of India, 2016].

An aging population is associated with an increase in the number of non communicable diseases like obesity, type2 diabetes mellitus [T2DM], hypertension, cardiovascular diseases, metabolic syndrome, and various types of cancer [Medhi GK, Mahanta J., 2007]. Obesity is considered a major risk factor for premature death and shortens the lifespan by 20 years [Reuser M, Bonneux L, Willekens F., 2008]. As one ages, there is progressive decrease in fat free mass (FFM or skeletal muscle), while fat mass reaches maximum levels at the age of 60 to 70. After the age of 70 FFM and body fat both tends to decrease, indicating that the redistribution of subcutaneous or body fat is associated with aging [Gallagher D, Visser M, De Meersman RE. et al., 1997]. Worldwide, a large volume of research is underway to investigate the relationship between aging and obesity, especially in an attempt to improve the quality of life.

However, all obese individuals do not exhibit the metabolic complications such individuals referred as metabolically healthy obesity (MHO) which is highly different from metabolically unhealthy obesity (MUHO) in terms of prevalence, etiology, pathogenesis, comorbidities and its related inflammatory patterns. It is interesting to note that 20% - 30 % of the adult obese population represents healthier metabolic profile without any complications known as MHO as compared to metabolically unhealthy obesity [Wildman RP., Muntner P, Reynolds K. et al., 2008]. A clear dissimilarity between metabolically healthy obesity (MHO) and metabolically unhealthy obesity (MUHO) has been reported in aged subjects as ageing population face the challenges of both rising number of the elderly and increasing obesity prevalence [Meigs JB, Lipinska I, Kathiresan S et al., 2007]. The MHO is highly prevalent in young age groups while MUHO is very common in elderly age groups that are why in depth metabolic phenotyping is required for different obesity phenotypes in the aged populations [Flegal KM, Carroll MD, Ogden CL. et al., 2002]. The phase transition from MHO to MUHO is dependent on various factors, including

Review of Literature

aging, levels of cytokine, adipokines and oxidative stress. Thus, it is important to study the initiating signals and regulatory downstream mechanisms involved in uncoupling of inflammatory signals during phase transitions from MHO to MUHO in different age groups.

2.5.2. Gender:

Overweight and obesity are linked with increased body weight due to excess energy intake and less physical activity. Gender is one of the essential factors that are affecting prevalence rate of obesity. Global survey data [Kanter R. and Caballero B., 2012] indicates that the prevalence rate of overweight and obesity among men and women varies by region and has risen rapidly from 1975 to 2015. In general, women tend to have higher prevalence rate for obesity (16 %) than males (12 %), whereas the prevalence of overweight is greater for males (24 %) than females (21 %). Kanter (2012) [Kanter R. and Caballero B., 2012] has further described that obesity was common in high income western countries in beginning of 1970s to 1980s but its prevalence increased in later years in low income and middle income countries.

Pattern of body fat distribution, adipose tissue storage, metabolism and sex hormones are main important factors responsible for gender differences. Females have higher percentage of body fat and have less free fatty mass than males of same BMI group, indicating the biological differences among them [Power ML and Schulkin J., 2008]. The gender wise disparity in prevalence rate is primarily associated with pattern of body fat distribution and adipose tissue storage. It is well known that sex hormones play a pivotal role in adipose tissue deposition, distribution, energy balance and metabolism especially female hormone estrogen which have both antioxidant and anti-inflammatory properties [Giordano S et al., 2015]. It has been reported that menopause affects body fat distribution that may increase the risk of weight gain (obesity) on health. It has also been reported that CuZn SOD, CAT decreased and MDA increased with increase in both age and body weight. The changes were more pronounced between premenstrual and postmenstrual groups than normally menstruating control and premenstrual group [Mittal PC. and Kant R., 2009]. It has been reported that menopause affects body fat distribution that may increase the risk of weight gain (obesity) on health. Weight gain as a function of age seems to be common among adults and obesity is more prevalent in women of middle and elder age group than young age group [Reuser M, Bonneux L, Willekens F., 2008; Pi-Sunyer FX., 1999]. Weight gain with menopause has been reported in several studies [Wing RR, Matthews KA, Kuller LH, et al., 1991; Pasquali R, Casimirri LF, Labate AMM, et al., 1995], the reason for which may be falling levels of estrogen [Yagi K., 1997; Ruiz-Larrea MB, Martin C, Martinez R, et al., 2000] which causes lowering of basal metabolic rate.

However, most studies in the field of obesity are related to metabolic complications in relation to age, gender and health status. As introduced earlier there is other phenotype of obesity characterized by favorable metabolic profile is known as metabolically healthy obesity (MHO). In contrast to metabolically unhealthy obesity, MHO individuals are also associated with adverse health consequences and to be found different in both genders [Onat A, Karadeniz Y, Tusun E. et al., 2016]. Therefore, in depth evaluation is required to investigate gender wise differences in different obesity phenotypes with regard to metabolic heath, oxidative stress and inflammation.

2.6. Pathophysiology associated with obesity:

From the foregoing, it is clear that obesity is a multifaceted health issue resulting from combination of multiple causes, and storage of surplus energy in adipose tissue is a major risk factor. Obesity is caused by complex etiological links between sedentary life style, quality and quantity of food intake, dietary patterns, medication use, genetic, endocrine, environmental factors etc. Moreover, it is associated with poor mental health condition and reduced quality of life. Obesity is also associated with mortality worldwide due to type 2 diabetes mellitus [T2DM], dyslipidemia, hypertension, metabolic syndrome, cardiovascular diseases and various type of cancer. It is therefore important to discuss the associations between obesity and various comorbidities.

2.6.1. Diabetes:

There is strong association between weight gain and diabetes in both genders and in all ethnic groups, which is why American Diabetes Association recommends clinical physicians to test for type 2 diabetes in overweight/obese people who are ≥45 years old, to assess the risk of future diabetes, and regardless of age, if they are morbid obese. Overweight raises the risk of type 2diabetes by 3 times and obesity by seven times compared to normal weight controls. [Abdullah A, Peeters A, de Courten M. et al., 2010]. Insulin resistance can be defined by loss of action of insulin, resulting in hyperinsulinaemia. Obesity is one of the major factor in development of type 2 diabetes because excess nutrient intake in form of free fatty acids, causing extension of adipose tissue mass. Free fatty acids (FFAs) decreases insulin sensitivity in muscles by preventing insulin mediated glucose uptake [Alberti KG and Zimmet PZ., 1998]. High level of blood glucose causes activation of insulin secretion by pancreas, resulting hyperinsulinemia. In the liver, FFAs increases the production of glucose triglycerides by the process of gluconeogenesis, glycogenesis, resulting the storage of excess glucose in form of glycogen and FFAs in the form of fat (triglyceride) in adipose tissues. In the presence of insulin resistance, higher amount of lipolysis of stored fat (triacylglycerol) molecules in adipose tissue yields more fatty acids, which can further prevent the anti-lipolytic effect of insulin, creating additional lipolysis in a vicious cycle [Bravata DM, Wells CK, Concato J et al., 2004].

2.6.2. Dyslipidaemia:

Obesity is also linked with altered lipid profile. Abnormalities in lipid metabolism related to obesity include, high low density of lipoprotein cholesterol (LDL-C), very low density of lipoprotein (VLDL), triglyceride (TG) and high serum cholesterol, as well as reduction in high density lipoprotein (HDL-C) [Grundy SM and Barnett JP., 1990]. The biochemical mechanism underlying obesity associated dyslipidaemia are not fully understood but involve the combination of hyperinsulinaemia and insulin resistance, resulting the stimulation of hepatic triglyceride synthesis in hypertrophic adipose tissue undergoing enhanced lipolysis. This will increase the concentration of postprandial hypertrigyceridaemia, LDL, and reduced HDL cholesterol concentrations and is an important criteria for diagnosis of dyslipidaemia [Eckel RH, Grundy SM, Zimmet et al., 2005].

2.6.3. Hypertension:

The relationship between weight gain and hypertension is well established. Adults represent linear relationship between weight gain in terms of body mass index (BMI) and blood pressure (BP), while weight loss reduces blood pressure in hypertensive respondents [Carmo JM, da Silva AA, Wang Z, et al., 2016]. In a 4-year follow-up study, conducted on 181 hypertensive overweight subjects, a 10 % weight loss was associated with 4.3/3.8 mmHg decrease in blood pressure, representing that weight loss is associated with anti-hypertensive effect [Schillaci G, Pasqualini L, Vaudo G., et al., 2003].

2.6.4. Metabolic Syndrome:

Metabolic syndrome is defined as clustering of metabolic risk components which include central obesity, type 2 diabetes mellitus, hypertension and dyslipidemia. Obesity is one of the most important risk factor for developing metabolic syndrome. Various clinical criteria have been developed to define metabolic syndrome. The definitions were proposed by several agencies such as the World Health Organization (WHO), the International Diabetes Federation (IDF) and that given by the National Institute of Health (NIH), USA. Of these, the simplest and the most widely accepted definition is that given by NIH in its third report of the National Cholesterol Education Program expert panel on detection, evaluation, and treatment of high blood cholesterol in adults. This report, known as the National Cholesterol Education Program's (NCEP) Adult Treatment Panel III (NCEP ATP III) 2002, modified in 2005, is as follows:

National Cholesterol Education Program's Adult Treatment Panel III (NCEP: ATP III) 2002: Individuals testing positive for any 3 out of the following 5 criteria are designated as suffering from MetS

- Central obesity: [waist circumference > 101 cm (male), > 88 cm (female)]

- Hyperglycemia: [Fasting plasma glucose ≥ 6.1 mmol/L, >100mg/dL]
- Hyper triglyceridaemia: [Triglycerides ≥ 1.7 mmol/L,>150 mg/Dl]
- HDL cholesterol: [Low HDL< 1.0 mmol/L, <40 mg/dL(male), < 1.3 mmol/L, <50 mg/dL (female)]
- Hypertension: [Blood Pressure ≥ 130/85 mm Hg or medication]

Central obesity increases the risk of metabolic abnormalities including metabolic syndrome and is translated into higher risk of all cause mortality compared to metabolically healthy normal weight individual.

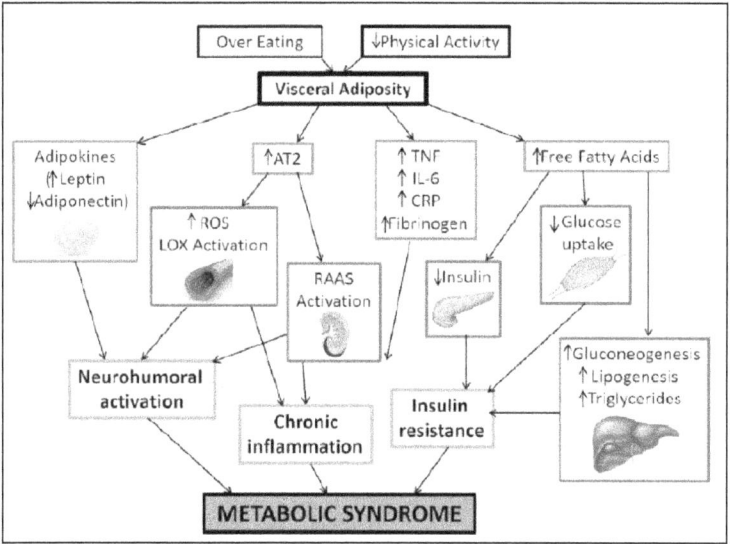

[Adopted from Y Rochlani et al., 2017]

Figure 2.2. Pathophysiological Mechanism in metabolically unhealthy obesity (MUHO) with Metabolic Syndrome

AT2, angiotensin II type 2 receptor; CRP, C-reactive protein; IL-6, interleukin 6; LOX, lectin-like oxidized low-density lipoprotein; RAAS, reninangiotensin-aldosterone system; ROS, reactive oxygen species; TNF, tumor necrosis factor.

The figure also summarizes the interrelationship among metabolically unhealthy obesity with metabolic syndrome (MUHO), oxidative stress and inflammation which is explained in the subsequent sections.

2.7. Role of Oxidative stress in obesity related diseases:

Oxidative stress is a condition which arises because the antioxidant defence system of the human body is not entirely efficient. Under these conditions increased free radical production is likely to lead to damage. In response to mild oxidative stress the body can increase its antioxidant defence levels [http://hdl.handle.net/10603/283028]. Unfortunately, toxin induced severe oxidative stress is capable of making free radicals or depleting antioxidant defence can lead to cell injury and death. There is evidence that free radical induced oxidative stress contributes to pathological conditions like obesity, diabetes and metabolic syndrome. It has been well established that systemic oxidative stress in adipose tissue leads to development of oxidative damage, triggering mitochondrial dysfunction, causing lipid accumulation and insulin resistance. [Bournat JC and Brown CW., 2010]. Imbalance in ROS levels triggers the irregular production of adipokines (decreased adiponectin and increased leptin secretion) associated with adipocyte dysfunction with impaired adipogenesis, that is, adipocyte hypertrophy [Wagner G, Lindroos-Christensen J, Einwallner E, et al., 2017]. One study showed that oxidative damage markers are higher in obese individuals and are directly correlated with percent body fat, BMI, LDL oxidation and TG levels [Pihl, E, Zilmer K, Kullisaar T et al., 2006]. The increased level of lipid peroxidation products (MDA), carbonylated proteins (PCO), nicotinamide adenine dinucleotide phosphate (NADPH)-oxidases (NOXs), and decreased antioxidants level namely catalase and glutathione (GSH) level were found in adipose tissue from obese individuals [Chattopadhyay M, Khemka VK, Chatterjee G et al., 2015]. It has been reported that body weight increases as age advances. It has been reported that menopause affects body fat distribution that may increase the risk of weight gain (obesity) on health. It has also been reported that SOD, CAT decreased and MDA increased with increase in both age and body weight. The changes were more pronounced between premenstrual and postmenstrual groups than normally menstruating control and premenstrual group [Mittal PC. and Kant R., 2009]. It has been also reported that menopause affects body fat distribution that may increase the risk of weight gain (obesity) on health.

These interactions and interrelationships between oxidative stress and obesity have been demonstrated in figure. 2.3.

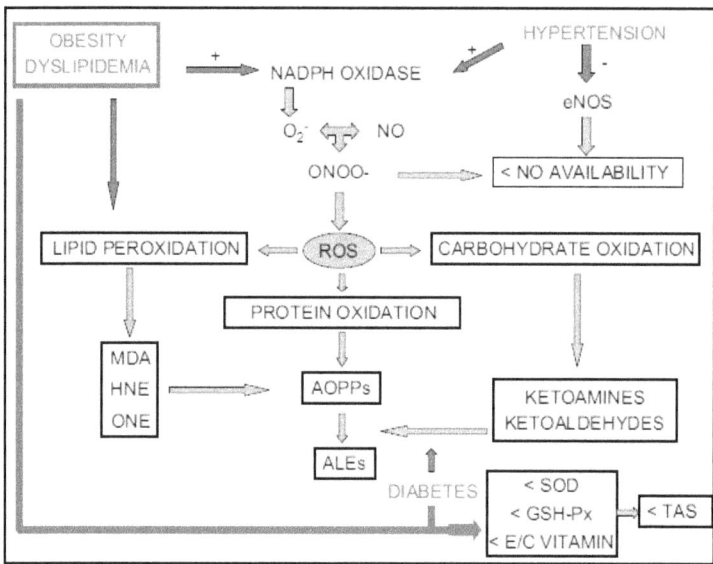

[Adopted from Hopps E et al., 2010]

Figure 2.3: Interrelationship between obesity and oxidative stress

2.8. Obesity and antioxidant capacity:

Oxygen is an essential element of life. When cells use oxygen to generate energy in the form of ATP (adenosine triphosphate) by mitochondria then ROS are produced as by product. These ROS species have dual role in living system depending upon their concentration. At low or moderate levels, ROS exhibit beneficial effects in living system; whereas at high level they induce oxidative stress, a deleterious process that can damage biomolecules. The effect of oxidative stress is countered by producing antioxidant enzymes which includes non-enzymatic and enzymatic antioxidants. In the antioxidant defence system, there is a chain of several antioxidants, scavenging property of one antioxidant may be followed by other. Interruption of oxidant/antioxidant balance in living system may cause pathological conditions that may cause obesity and other metabolic complications. In a previous study, it has been shown that the obese individuals have lower level of antioxidant enzymes such as superoxide dismutase (SOD) and catalase (CAT), and glutathione peroxidase (GPx) compared to healthy persons [Ozata, M., Mergen, M., Oktenli, C. et al., 2002]. GPx is selenoenzyme, which catalyzes the degradation of hydrogen peroxide and hydroperoxides at the expense of glutathione. It has been reported that GPx, CuZn-SOD, and CAT activities were reduced in red blood cells (RBCs) of obese women when compared with normal weight non obese group [Amirkhizi F, Siassi F, Minaie S et al., 2007]. Lower GSH/GSSG ratio in animal models of obesity have also been reported [Foster MW, McMahon TJ, Stamler JS et al., 2003].

2.9. Oxidative stress and mechanisms of cellular damage: role of free radicals

Oxidative stress is generally described as a disturbance in the balance between reactive oxygen/nitrogen species (ROS/RNS) and body's antioxidant capacity, resulting in the accumulation of toxic free radical species that can cause direct or indirect effect on different biomolecules and organs [Vincent HK, Innes KE, Vincent KR., 2007].

Free radicals defined as a species, which is capable of independent existence that contains one or more unpaired electrons, that is alone in orbital [Halliwell B, 1989]. Most biological molecules are non radicals, which contains only paired electrons. Because electrons are more stable when paired together in orbitals, thus radicals are more reactive than non radical species. Radicals react with other molecules in various ways [Slater TF, 1984]. For example, if two radicals join, they can combine their unpaired electrons and form a covalent bond.

In order to pair, a radical might donate its unpaired electron to another molecule, or it might take an electron from another molecule. However, if a radical gives or takes one electron from a non radical, that non radical becomes a radical. One radical begets another and so on. Some examples of free radicals are given below:

a) Oxygen centered free radicals (ROS): ($O2^{\cdot -}$) Superoxide, ($OH^{\cdot}$) Hydroxyl, ($ROO^{\cdot}$) Peroxyl radicals

b) Nitrogen centered free radicals: ($NO^{\cdot}$) Nitric oxide, (NO_2) Nitrogen dioxide radicals.

There are two important sources of ROS generation in the biological system:

a) Environmental: Drugs, pesticides, tobacco, alcohol, radiations, high temperature (Hemnani and Parihar, 1998)

b) Cellular metabolism: Mitochondrial electron transport, endoplasmic reticulum enzyme activities, prostaglandin synthesis, activated phagocytic cells etc. [Cheeseman KH and Slater TF., 1993].

2.9.1. Oxidative damage to lipids:

Membrane lipids present in sub cellular organelles are highly susceptible to free radical damage. Lipids when react with the free radicals, can undergo highly damaging chain reactions leading to both direct and indirect effects. The oxidative deterioration of membrane lipids is known as lipid peroxidation (LPO) [Slater TF., 1983]. This results in production of a chemical species called lipid hydroperoxides (Fig 2.3). These lipid hydroperoxides care then degraded to a variety of products including alkenals, hydroalkenals, ketones, alkanes etc [Logani and Davies., 1980].

LPO can be estimated by the detection of conjugated dienes formed during the early phase of peroxidation and less commonly by the measurement of lipid hydroperoxides [Rexknagel RO and Glende EA., 1984]. The most common procedures are based on the measurement of the products of lipid peroxidation breakdown such as malondialdehyde (MDA) [Esterbauer H, Lang J, Zadravee S et al., 1984]. MDA reacts with biological substances to form Schiff's base, which may be assayed fluorometrically [Dillard CJ and Tappel AL., 1984]. LPO has also been assayed by the evolution of short chain alkanes, i.e., ethane and pentane, both in vitro and in vivo [Muller A and Sies H., 1984]. The pathway for the production of MDA via LPO has been outlined in figure 2.3.

The process of LPO consists of three stages: initiation, propagation and termination. Peroxyl radicals (ROO) once formed can be rearranged via a cyclization reaction to endoperoxides (precursors of malondialdehyde) and the final product of the peroxidation process is MDA. Another major aldehydic product of LPO besides MDA is 4 hydroxy-2-nonetal (HNE). MDA is mutagenic in bacterial and mammalian cells and is carcinogenic in rats. HNE is weakly mutagenic but it can be the major toxic product of LPO. Moreover, HNE has strong effects on the phenotypic characteristics of the cells. LPO is an autocatalytic process, which can be terminated by the recombination of radicals or depletion of the radicals.

The unsaturated fatty acids present in membranes (phospholipids, glycolipids, glycerides and sterols) and the transmembrane proteins containing oxidizable amino acids are susceptible to free radical damage. Also, increased membrane permeability caused by LPO or oxidation of structurally important proteins can cause breakdown of transmembrane ion gradient, loss of secretory function and inhibition of integrated cellular metabolic processes. The free radicals derived from PUFA can also abstract hydrogen atoms from membrane proteins and –SH containing enzymes are particularly susceptible. The amino acid radicals thus generated can form disulphide bridges, protein lipid and protein-protein covalent bonds. The cross- linking of proteins inactivates enzymes and produces high molecular weight fluorescent aggregates known as ceroid, lipofuscein or age pigments. MDA can also cross link the amino group of phosphatidyl ethanolamine molecule, phosphatidyl serine or proteins, disturbing the membrane structure [Beneditti A, Comporti M, Fulceri R. et al., 1984]. The cell surfaces are capable of serving as both targets of ROS and as a gate that provides a barrier to charged species and can also modify other radical species to a more permeable and reactive form. Free radicals can attack may depend on the product solubility and the by product diffusion distances. OH^- have a high indiscriminate reactivity, so this free radical is not likely to diffuse away from cellular site of production and may react nearby. Less reactive free radicals may be capable of reacting distally from the sites of generation. H2O2 has been shown to diffuse across biological membranes, mitochondrial membrane and peroxisome membrane, thus potentially exerting toxic effects at a distance from its site of generation [Turrens JF., Freeman BA., Levitt JG. et al., 1982].

2.9.2. Oxidative damage to Proteins:

The ionizing radiation studies have demonstrated that when proteins reacts with OH it leads to the formation of carbon centered radical and a hydrogen atom is absorbed from the proteins peptide back bone, this carbon centered radical under aerobic conditions reacts readily with dioxygen to form peroxyl radicals which is further then converted to the alkyl peroxides by reactions with the protonated form of superoxide (HO_2) [Stadtman,ER., 2004]. In the absence of ionizing radiations, the same reaction can be initiated by OH produced by the Fenton reaction under in vivo conditions. Thus, when radiations are not present, the proteins are resistant to damage by H_2O_2 and other minor oxidants provided no transition metal is present. Metal catalyzed damage to proteins involves oxidation of proteins by loss of histidine residues, introduction of carbonyl groups and the formation of protein centered alkyl (R), alkoxyl (RO) and alkylperoxy (ROO) radicals.

The oxidation of proteins by ROS results in the formation of different kinds of inter and intra protein crosslinkages. Cysteine and methionine residues are most susceptible to oxidation of ROS. Almost all forms of ROS are able to oxidize methionine residues of proteins to methionine residues of proteins serves as an important antioxidant function to protect cells from oxidative damage. It has been proved by many studies in animal models that the process of ageing is often associated with the accumulation of oxidized form of proteins [Stadtman,ER., 2001]. The accumulation of of oxidized proteins in living systems can be due to an organism. The decrease in the ability to degrade oxidized proteins due to either decrease in the protease concentrations and/or to an increased level of protease inhibitors may be other reasons of increased ROS.

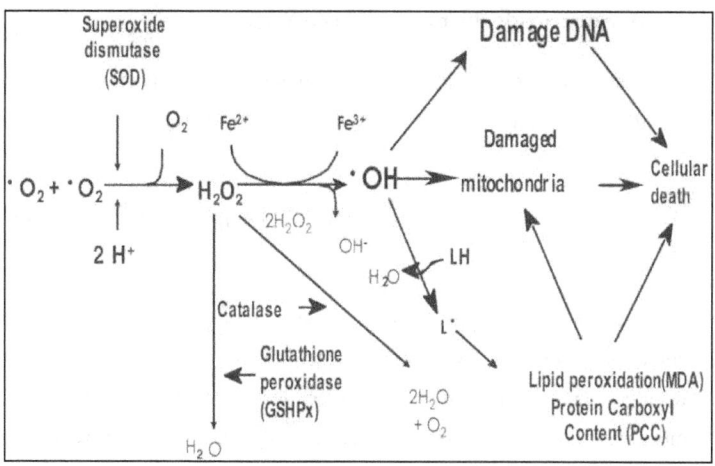

Figure 2.4: Mechanism of Oxidative Stress in cellular damage

2.10. Antioxidant defence mechanisms in the cells:

The effect of free radicals is counteracted by the enzymatic as well as non enzymatic antioxidants. These antioxidants defences are important as they directly remove the oxidants (free radicals). Antioxidants specifically quench the free radicals, chelate redox metals or interact with other antioxidants and regenerate them. Antioxidants should be readily absorbed and must have a concentration in tissues and body fluids at physiological relevant level, to work in the aqueous and/or lipid phase. Some of the most effective enzymatic antioxidants are superoxide dismutase (SOD), catalase (CAT), and glutathione peroxidase (GSH-Px). Non enzymatic antioxidants involve thiol antioxidants (glutathione, thioredoxin and lipoic acid), vitamin C, vitamin E, carotenoids, polyphenols, melatonin etc. Vitamin C reacts with O_2 in the aqueous phase, while vitamin E reacts with O_2 in the lipophilic phase. Some of the antioxidants can generate other antioxidants and thus restore their original function. This process is called as antioxidants network [Sies H., Stahl W., Sevanian A., 2005]. The redox cycle of vitamin C and vitamin E forms such an antioxidant network. The capacity to generate one antioxidant by another is driven by the redox potentials of the [Red/Ox]. It has been seen in many studies that there is link between increased levels of ROS and disturbed activities of enzymatic and non enzymatic antioxidants in cells.

2.10.1. Superoxide dismutase (CuZn SOD)

SOD is a class of closely related enzymes that catalyze the breakdown of the superoxide anion into oxygen and hydrogen peroxide [Zelko IN, Mariani TJ, Folz RJ., 2002].

$Cu^{2+}\text{-SOD} + 2\ O \rightarrow Cu^{+}\text{-SOD} + O_2$ $Cu^{2+}\text{-SOD} + 2\ O + 2H^+ \rightarrow Cu^{2+}\text{-SOD} + H_2O_2$

There are several isoforms of SOD, differing in the nature of active metal centre and amino acid constituency as well as their number of subunits, cofactors and other features. In humans, there are three forms of SOD: cytosolic CuZn SOD; mitochondrial Mn SOD: and extracellular SOD (EC-SOD). SOD quenches O_2 with high reaction rates by successive oxidation and reduction of the transition metal ion at the active site in a ping pong type mechanism.

CuZn SOD is a homodimer having a molecular weight of 32 KDa. Each subunit contains an active site of dinuclear metal cluster constituted by copper and zinc ions. Mitochondrial Mn SOD is a homotetramer of 96 KDa containing one of the most effective antioxidant enzymes also having anti tumor activity. Studies on different cell lines have confirmed that over expression of Mn SOD leads to tumor growth radiation. Extracellular SOD (EC-SOD) is a secretory, tetrameric, copper and zinc containing glycoprotein present in fluids and ha high affinity for certain glycosaminoglycans such as heparin and heparin sulphate. Its regulation occurs primarily in a manner coordinated by cytokines, rather than a response of individual cells to the oxidant in mammalian tissues.

2.10.2. Catalase:

Catalase is present in plants, animals and aerobic bacteria. It is located in the peroxisome. The enzyme decomposes H_2O_2 to water and molecular oxygen. Catalase has one of the highest turnover rates for all enzymes: one molecule of catalase can convert 6 million molecules of H_2O_2 to water and oxygen per minute [Valko M, Leibfritz D, Moncol J et al., 2007].

$2H_2O_2 \rightarrow 2H_2O + O_2$

CAT is abundant in liver and erythrocytes. The usual form of CAT consists of four protein subunits each containing a haem (Fe^{3+} protoporphyrin) group bound to its active site. The dissociation of subunits results in its loss of activity. The inhibitors of CAT include azide, cyanide. 3 amino 1,2, 4 trizole, reduced glutathione and dithiothreitol. The significantly decreased capacity to detoxify H_2O_2 is associated with decreased level of catalase in a variety of tumors [Valko M, Leibfritz D, Moncol J et al. 2007].

2.10.3. Glutathione peroxidase (GPx):

There are two forms of the enzymes GSH-Px, one is Se independent, while the other is Se dependent GSH-Px. They differ in the number of subunits, the bonding nature of Se at the active centre and their catalytic mechanisms. Se dependent GSH-Px is a tetramer. It contains one residue of selenocysteine per mole at each of the active sites and is found in cytosol (70%) and mitochondria (30 %). Cyanide and superoxide radicals inhibit GSH-Px [Blum J., and Fridovich I., 1985]. All GSH-Px enzymes, add two electrons to reduce peroxides by forming selenoles (Se-OH). The antioxidant properties of these selenoenzymes allow them to eliminate peroxides, which can be potential substrate for the fenton reaction. Reaction involving iron and hydrogen peroxides, which is capable of oxidizing a wide range of substrates and cause biological damage, is referred as the Fenton reaction. It is complex and capable of generating both hydroxyl radicals and higher oxidation states of iron. GSH-Px acts in conjugation with GSH, which is present in cells at high concentrations. H_2O_2 or an organic peroxide (ROOH) are the substrate for the catalytic reaction of GSH-Px. GSH-Px decomposes peroxides to water (or alcohol) and simultaneously oxidizing GSH.

The main reaction that glutathione peroxidase catalyzes is:

$2GSH + H_2O_2 \rightarrow GS\text{–}SG + 2H_2O$

Where GSH represents reduced monomericglutathione, and GS-SG represents glutathione disulfide.

2.10.4. Non-enzymatic defence:

In non enzymatic defence antioxidants such as vitamin E, lipoic acid, L arginine, β carotene and coenzyme Q are present within cell membranes. The lipophilic vitamin E is a highly effective antioxidant, it directly acts on peroxyl radicals and inhibit the propagation of peroxyl free radicals in tissues, by reacting them to form a vit E or tocopheryl radical which will then be oxidized by hydrogen donor (vit c) and then return to its reduced state

2.10.5. FRAP Assay:

The total antioxidant capacity known as the ferric reducing ability of plasma (FRAP). This is a measure of the total antioxidant capacity of plasma, based on the reduction of ferrous ions by the effect of the reducing power ability of plasma constituents, and contributed by low molecular weight antioxidants of a hydrophilic and hydrophobic character such as Vitamin C, Vitamin E, bilirubin and uric acid [Benzie IF and Strain JJ., 1996]. The low molecular weight compounds are vitamin c, vitamin E, bilirubin and uric acid. FRAP is good biochemical marker which give more accurate information regarding total antioxidant than that provided by individual antioxidant measurements and which may describe the dynamic equilibrium between pro-oxidant and antioxidants in the plasma.

Plasma contains low molecular weight compounds like Vitamin C, Vitamin E, bilirubin and uric acid that possess antioxidant properties. The total antioxidant capacity known as the ferric reducing ability of plasma (FRAP) is a measure of the antioxidant power, on the basis of reduction of ferric ions to ferrous ions by the effect of the reducing power of plasma constituents [Benzie I F and Strain J.J., 1996]. FRAP is supposed to provide more biological information than that given by individual antioxidant measurements and can explain the dynamic equilibrium of pro-oxidants and antioxidants in the plasma.

2.11. Obesity and inflammation:

Inflammation is an ordered sequence of physiological response of the organism against harmful stimuli to maintain systemic metabolic homeostasis. Obesity is associated with chronic low grade inflammation by the activation of inflammatory response in metabolically dynamic organ such as insulin sensitive tissues, particularly adipose tissue [Karalis KP, Giannogonas P, Kodela E et al., 2009]. However, obesity increases the stress response by impairment of the inflammation process. This response is characterized by increasing levels of renin angiotensin aldosterone system, glucorticoids (steroid hormone) and needed for the development and differentiation adipocyte stem cells. In addition, there is sharp increase in blood proinflammatory markers, adipokines and cytokines with increasing adiposity [Karalis KP, Giannogonas P, Kodela E., et al., 2009]. In this context, adipose tissue secrete one of the major contributor of inflammation tumor necrosis factor alpha (TNF-α), Interleukin (IL 6), C reactive protein (CRP), monocytes chemotactic protein -1, plasminogen activator inhibitor 1 (PAI-1) or resistin in obese state supported the relationship between obesity and inflammation [Kintscher U, Hartge M, Hess K., et al., 2008]. Dysregulated secretion of adipokines from adipose tissue is responsible for obesity associated metabolic complications.

2.11.1. Tumor Necrosis Factor- alpha (TNF- α) and Obesity:

TNF- α is one of the important pro inflammatory adipokine linked to obesity, insulin resistance, metabolic syndrome, secreted by monocyte macrophages from the vascular stroma, particularly M1 macrophages, and endothelial cells, particularly in the visceral adipocytes of obese subjects. TNF- α has been considered an essential adipokines that link obesity to insulin resistance [Schmidt MI, Duncan BB, Sharrett AR et al., 1999]. Several studies have shown that the level of TNF- α and its messenger RNA (m RNA) positively correlated with body fat, BMI and decrease in obese subjects with weight loss. TNF- α induces the obesity mediated insulin resistance via phosphorylation of serine residue at c-Jun NH2-terminal kinase of insulin receptor 1 (IRS-1) that has an inhibitory effect on insulin signalling [Balistreri CR, Caruso C, Candore G., 2010]. In addition, TNF- α inhibits the activity of lipoprotein lipase (LPL) and increase the mobilization of fatty acids from adipose tissue to blood stream [Hermsdorff HH, Zulet MA, Bressan J., et al., 2008]. Increased level of TNF- α induces the activation of nuclear factor kappa B (NF-κB) pathway which increases the expression of IL 6, chemokines (C-C motif) ligand 2 (CCL2) and decreasing the expression of adiponectin [Lee J., 2013].

2.11.2. Interleukin 6 (IL 6) and Obesity:

IL 6 is a proinflammatory cytokine that is involved in normal inflammatory response against infection, tissue injury and inflammation. Approximately, one third of circulating IL 6 secreted by M 1 macrophage of adipose tissue. Adipocyte hypertrophy and inflammatory stimuli such as tumor necrosis factor alpha, induces the production of IL 6 which further activate the cell signalling pathways, including m TOR and protein kinase C (PKC) to induce insulin resistance. This occurs primarily in visceral adipose tissues, indicating the positive correlation between obesity and insulin resistance [Maury E, Brichard SM., 2010].

The mechanism of action of IL 6 with insulin resistance are similar to those reported for TNF occurring from inhibition of lipoprotein lipase and phosphorylation of serine residue of insulin receptor. In addition, IL 6 induces the production of C reactive protein (CRP) in the liver, and has been linked to obesity associated hypertriglyceridemia by stimulating the secretion of very low density lipoprotein (VLDL) from liver to blood stream [Leal V de O, Mafra D., 2013].

2.11.3. C reactive protein (CRP) and Obesity:

The C reactive protein (CRP) is acute marker of inflammation which is synthesized by hepatic cells in the presence of IL 6 and known to increase in circulation in response to tissue injury, infection and inflammation [Pradhan AD, Manson JE, Rifai N, et al., 2001]. CRP is standardized marker of cardiovascular diseases. CRP is major downstream mediator of acute phase response responsible for sequential inflammatory event. CRP is chief acute marker responsible for complement system leading to the opsonisation through activation of C1q molecule. It can also initiate fluid phase pathway followed by cell mediated pathway in the presence of host defence by activating complement as well as to binding to Fc receptors of IgG [Pradhan AD, Manson JE, Rifai N et al., 2001]. Interaction between Fc receptors of IgG and CRP, leading to the release of proinflammatory cytokines [Du Clos TW. 2000]. CRP levels are strongly associated with insulin resistance, dyslipidemia, and with levels of the pro-inflammatory cytokines, IL-6, and TNF-α. Furthermore Insulin Resistance and Atherosclerosis Study (IRAS) showed that hs-CRP was positively correlated with BMI, waist circumference, and fasting insulin and inversely correlated with HDL cholesterol (HDL-C) and insulin sensitivity index. The strongest associations were observed between CRP levels, central adiposity, and insulin resistance.

From the foregoing, it is clear that oxidative stress and inflammation are interconnected to each other and to obesity and its associated comorbidities. The rise in level of both oxidative stress and inflammation sets up a vicious cycle in obesity and its related complications [Gao M, Lv J, Yu C., et al., 2020]. This group of obese is designated Metabolically Unhealthy Obesity (MUHO).

However, as described earlier, recent studies have identified a group of obese who do not display biochemical abnormalities associated with metabolic syndrome. These have been designated as a phenotype known as Metabolically Healthy Obesity (MHO). None of the studies discussed above have investigated these associations in this group.

There is some evidence that an increase in oxidative stress and inflammation induced by it plays an important role in the transition of MHO to MUHO with metabolic syndrome or other complications [Gao M, Lv J, Yu C., et al., 2020] even as studies are lacking which establish the temporal sequence of the relationship. Obesity is a multifaceted health issue resulting from combination of multiple causes but storage of surplus energy in adipose tissue is a major risk factor. Excess nutrient intake can trigger signaling responses in one organ or tissue. Many cell types give rise to metabolic dysfunction.

In addition to obesity, there is another intermediate state designated as overweight. Again, based on the National Cholesterol Education Program's (NCEP) Adult Treatment Panel III (NCEP ATP III) 2002, modified in 2005, some among the overweight group maybe at risk to develop metabolic syndrome, designated Metabolically Unhealthy Overweight (MUHOw), while others show a healthy metabolic profile and are designated Metabolically Healthy Overweight (MHOw). Data which compares these groups for NCEP: ATP III risk factors for metabolic syndrome, oxidative stress markers and redox balance and inflammatory indices is lacking.

These are important questions which require investigation to understand the phenotype known as Metabolically Healthy, which may comprise of normal weight, overweight and obese groups with regard to their NCEP ATP III risk factors for metabolic syndrome, oxidative stress markers and redox balance, and inflammatory indices. The present study has been designed to investigate these groups.

The next question that arises in conduct of any investigation is its design. The investigations to understand the interrelationships in human disease have often centered on animal models because these are easier to control for individual variables such as age and gender, and can be studied in more invasive ways. Hence, another issue in any research study is that of the choice of research model.

Creation of the obesity in animal models has employed high fat diet induced, chemical induced methods and use of genetic models. Methodologies include high-fat feeding studies, which require only a few months to induce Obesity. There are several spontaneously occurring obese mouse strains that have also been used for decades and that are very well characterized. Animal models have been used because they allow data collection in controlled conditions, with minimization of inter individual variations. Among animals, rats are most popular because of the ease in maintaining them, but subtle and obvious differences between humans and rat models in terms of anatomy, physiology and cellular metabolism make it complicated to apply research data derived from rat and other animal studies to human conditions, and accurately translating information from rat studies can be an exercise involving assumptions that may be questionable.

Therefore, for the present study, the human model was selected for better understanding of a realistic in vivo scenario, since there is no known animal model for metabolically healthy obesity.

Different type of research designs are used in human studies. In epidemiology, meta-analysis, systemic review, practice guidelines, randomized control trial, cohort study, case control study, case report are some examples. To study the effect of obesity indices on oxidative stress markers, antioxidant balance and inflammatory markers, we have adopted case control design for the following reasons: Case control studies are observational because no intervention is attempted and no attempt is made to alter the course of the disease. The goal is to retrospectively determine the exposure to the risk factor of interest from each of the two groups of individuals: cases and controls.

The only tissue that can be conveniently obtained from humans in clinical studies is blood, which is routinely used by clinicians and researchers for assaying various diagnostic markers like oxidative stress and inflammatory markers in serum, plasma and erythrocytes.

Hence all the studies in the present investigation have been conducted using blood samples and findings have been related to non-invasive measures such as body mass index and waist circumference

Based on these issues, the present study was conducted on metabolically healthy non obese controls, and their overweight and obese counterparts to measure cause-effect relationships with regard to age, gender, body fat distribution, oxidative stress and inflammatory markers.

Chapter-3

METHODS AND MATERIALS

3.1. Selection criteria for detection of metabolically healthy obesity (MHO):

Metabolically healthy obesity (MHO) is a unique subset of obese phenotype which is described by absence of metabolic syndrome. Although there are no universal classification criteria to define MHO but the NCEP ATP III criteria [NCEP ATP III, 2005] for diagnosing metabolic syndrome is the most acceptable in clinical practice. According to NCEP ATP III criteria, participants suffering from any three of the following Met S risk factors namely, Central obesity (waist circumference ≥ 102 cm/40 inches (male), ≥ 88 cm/35 inches (female), Hyperglycaemia ≥ 110 mg/dl), Dyslipidemia (TG ≥ 150 mg/dl, HDL-C < 40 mg/dL (male), < 50 mg/dL (female)) and Blood pressure $\geq 130/85$ mmHg (or treated for hypertension) are designated MetS. The conglomerate of these risk factors have been designated as Met S risk factors and have been measured for all respondents to confirm that they are metabolically healthy. They have been quantitatively analyzed for all objectives. Thus, respondents who represent the absence of metabolic syndrome risk factors were included in the study and are termed as Metabolically Healthy Obesity (MHO).

3.2. Selection of Respondents:

The study was conducted on persons visiting outpatient departments (OPDs) of government hospitals such as Beli Hospital, Swaroop Rani Nehru Hospital, Kamala Nehru Memorial Hospital and private pathologies in Allahabad, India, during the years 2015 to 2017. They were screened for inclusion and exclusion criteria.

3.3. Inclusion Criteria:

According to NCEP ATP III definition, persons not suffering from any of the following risk factors, namely, Dyslipidemia (TG ≥ 150 mg/dl, HDL-C< 40 mg/dL (male), < 50 mg/dL (female)] and Blood pressure ≥ 130/85 mmHg (or treated for hypertension) and Fasting plasma glucose ≥ 110 mg/dl) were included in the study and are termed 'Metabolically Healthy (MH)'.

3.4. Exclusion criteria:

Those who had been diagnosed by a physician as suffering from other metabolic conditions, any infectious disease, neurological disease or malignancy etc. were excluded. Those younger than 20 years and older than 80 years were also excluded.

All those who satisfied the inclusion and exclusion criteria were designated as **Metabolically Healthy (MH)**.

The significance of the study was explained to all MH respondents and they were requested to give about 6 ml of blood. Those who gave their informed consent were enrolled for the study. The study protocol was approved vide office order no. **IERB/2016/03** by the Institutional Ethics Committee of Population Resource & Research Centre, Allahabad. Finally, 349 respondents who fulfilled all inclusion and exclusion criteria and consented to participate in the study were enrolled.

3.5. Study Design:

The present study was conducted on Indian metabolically healthy adults aged 20 to 80 years to assess the impact of their body mass index on selected biochemical indices of Met S risk factors, oxidative stress, redox balance, and inflammatory markers.

We adopted the case control design because they are observational studies where no intervention is attempted and no attempt is made to alter the course of the disease. The goal is to retrospectively determine the exposure to the risk factor of interest from each of the two groups of individuals: Cases and Controls.

3.6. Further assessment of the individuals who fulfilled inclusion and exclusion criteria:

3.6.1 Measurement of Body Mass Index and waist circumference:

The height and weight of all metabolically healthy respondents were measured following standard procedures, as recommended by WHO [WHO, 1995]. Body mass index (BMI) was calculated as BMI = weight (kg)/ [height (m)]^2. Their waist circumference (WC) was measured using flexible measuring tape at the natural waistline above the umbilicus and below the rib cage and recorded in centimeters (cm).

3.6.2 Division of respondents into Study groups:

In Chapters 1-3, the main objective of the study was to compare Metabolically Healthy Non-obese (MHNO), Metabolically Healthy Overweight (MHOw) and Metabolically Healthy Obese (MHO) respondents.

The currently most accepted criteria for this division is as described by WHO guidelines [WHO, 1995] which categorizes adult obesity into three different grades, (i) Non obese controls: BMI≤25 kg/m^2 (ii) Overweight: 25-30 kg/m^2 (iii) Obese BMI>30 kg/m^2. Based on this, the respondents were categorized as follows:

(a) Metabolically healthy non obese (MHNO, N=100), (b) Metabolically healthy overweight (MHO$_W$, N=147), (c) Metabolically healthy obese (MHO, N=102). Care was taken to enroll approximately equal number of males and females in all groups.

Even as this WHO criteria is the most commonly used, the Indian Consensus Group for Asian Indians [Misra A, 2015] have recommended revised guidelines for Asians, particularly Indians, to divide the non-obese group according to the WHO criteria into two groups, a BMI of ≥ 23 kg/m^2 and ≥ 25 kg/m^2 as overweight and obese respectively.

Hence, Chapter 1 has been divided into two sections, A and B. **In Section A**, the respondents have been grouped by the WHO criteria into MHNO, MHOw and MHO. **In Section B**, the guidelines for Asian Indians have been used for classification, and compared with the groups in Section A. Results from this comparison were used to decide which criteria is more appropriate for use in other chapters.

In Chapter 4, the metabolically healthy (MH) respondents have been categorized into three groups; MH Non-obese controls (BMI<25, waist circumference <90 cm), and those with General Obesity (MHGO) or those with Central Obesity (MHCO), based on their waist circumference, non-obese and those suffering from was compared with General Obesity (GO) (BMI$\geq$25, waist circumference < 90 cm (males), <80 cm (females)), and Central Obesity (CO) (BMI>25, waist circumference $\geq$ 90 cm (males), $\geq$ 80 cm (females) [WHO, 2008].

In Chapter 5, the MHO group of 102 respondents was as described above and was compared with a group called Metabolically Unhealthy Obese (MUHO) of 102 respondents. The data for MUHO was taken from a co-worker of my lab because it was important to obtain this was an important question pertaining to public health. MUHO comprised of metabolically unhealthy obese respondents, with metabolic syndrome, who were suffering from all five risk factors of MetS as prescribed by NCEP ATP III, that is Central obesity, High Fasting plasma glucose, High Blood pressure (or treated for hypertension), Dyslipidemia (TG $\geq$ 150 mg/dl, HDL-C < 40 mg/dL (male) (DL), < 50 mg/dL (female)). The final sample comprised of n=102, comprising 62 males and 40 females.

Cross sectional case control study: Chapters 1-3

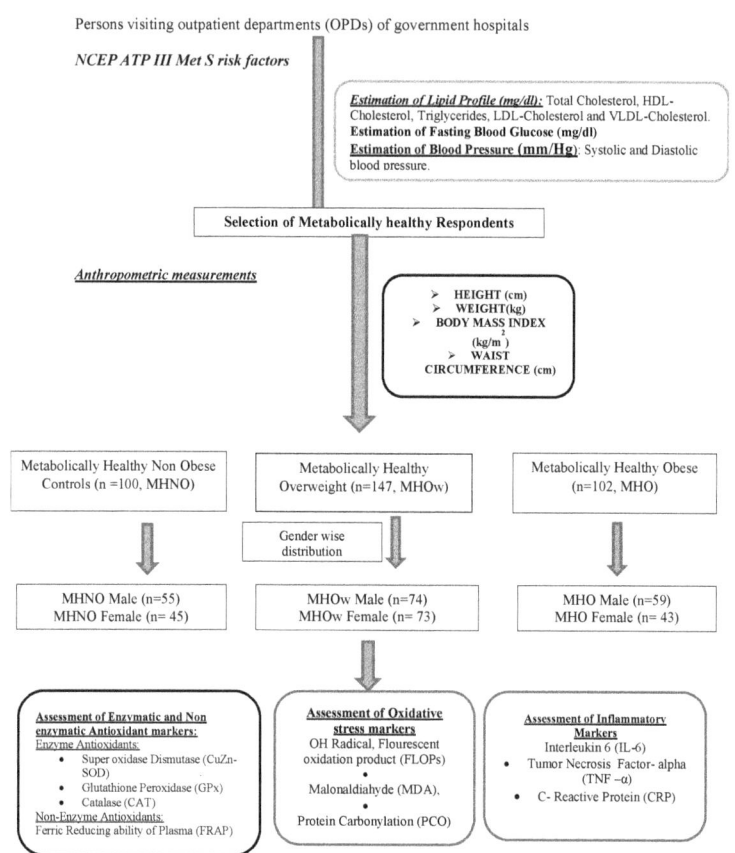

Figure 3.1. Flowchart for the selection and distribution of respondents for Chapters 1-3.

3.7. Blood Collection, Processing and Storage:

At each blood collection, 6 ml of fasting venous blood was drawn. All samples were collected in the morning in order to avoid any confounding effect of diurnal variation of parameters.1 ml of blood was withdrawn into an EDTA vial for estimation of Hemoglobin (Hb) and 3 ml of blood was withdrawn into Acid-Citrate-Dextrose (ACD) vials for isolation of plasma and RBCs and kept on ice for not more than 1 hour after processing. Remaining 2 ml of blood were withdrawn in plain vial for collection of serum. After centrifugation of whole blood at 3000 rpm for 5 min, serum from plain vial, and plasma and red blood cells (RBCs) from anticoagulant vials were collected. Serum and plasma aliquots were packed in sample tubes and stored. Plasma and serum were transferred into separate tubes and stored at - 80°C, until analysis.

3.8. Preparation of erythrocyte lysate:

Collected red blood cells (RBCs) were washed three times with normal saline. RBC was used to prepare 1:20 hemolysate. Packed RBCs obtained were suspended in approximately 1 volume of 0.154 M NaCl. To 0.2 ml of this suspension, 1.8 ml of β-merceptoethanol-EDTA stabilizing solution (0.05 ml of β-merceptoethanol and 10 ml of neutralized 10% EDTA in distilled water was added. 1:20 hemolysate were transferred into separate tubes and stored at - 80°C, until analysis.

3.9. Estimation of Haemoglobin (Hb):

Haemoglobin in blood was estimated by Drabkin solution. 5 ml of Drabkin solution was added to 0.02 ml of blood and absorbance was recorded after 10 min at 540 nm against a Drabkin reagent blank in spectrophotometer. Hb was expressed as g/dl of blood.

3.10. Fasting Blood Glucose and Lipid profile:

The measurements of lipid profile parameters and fasting blood glucose were estimated using the standard autoanalyser kits manufactured by ERBA diagnostics Mannheim, Germany. The LDL cholesterol was calculated using the Friedewald formula: $LDL\text{-}C = TC - HDL\text{-}C - (TG/5)$ .and $VLDL = (TG/5)$.

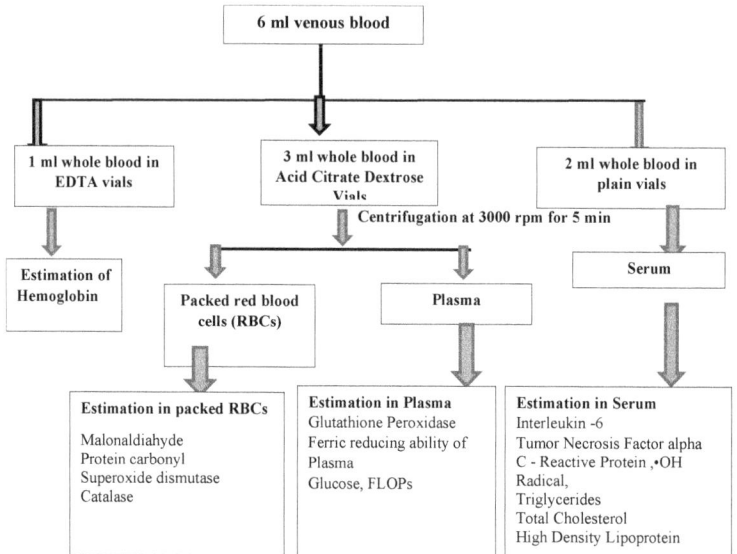

Figure 3.2. Flowchart for processing of blood and fractions used for biochemical estimations.

3. 11 Assessment of Oxidative Stress Markers

3.11.1 Hydroxyl radicals ($^{•}OH$):

The spectrofluorometric analysis of ($^{•}OH$) radicals was done by following the protocol described by Korotkova and Bashkim et al (2011) with slight modifications. To evaluate the ($^{•}OH$) radicals in plasma/serum, a non-fluorescent terephallic acid (TA) hydroxylated into a brilliant fluorophore into 2 hydroxyterephallic acid (TA-OH) in the presence of ($^{•}OH$) radicals. To investigate the quantity of hydroxyl radicals in serum, 2 ml of 10^{-2} mol/L terephalate solution, 2 ml of phosphate buffer (0.025 M, pH 6.8) and 0.5 ml of serum samples were added into the 10 ml cell. The fluorescence intensity was measured at 327/315 nm wavelength (excitation/emission) by using cary eclipse fluorescence spectrophotometer (Agilent technologies).

3.11.2 Fluorescent Oxidation Products (FLOPs):

The procedure for measuring fluorescent oxidation products (FLOP) were adapted from the modified method of Tianying et al., (2004). In brief, 0.2 ml of plasma samples was mixed with 1 ml of ethanol/ether (3:1 v/v) and centrifuged at 3000 rpm, after which supernatant was added to cuvettes for spectrofluorometric readings. The fluorescence can be determined as relative fluorescence intensity units per mililiter of plasma at 360/430 nm wavelength (excitation/emission) by a fluorometer (cary eclipse fluorescence spectrophotometer, Agilent technologies).

3.11.3 Malondialdehyde (MDA):

Malondialdehyde (MDA) is an index for lipid peroxidation, and estimated in erythrocytic hemolysate, a method described by Niehaus & Samuelsson et al., (1968). 0.3 ml of hemolysate was mixed with 0.8 ml of 0.1 M phosphate buffer (pH 7.4), and 2 ml of 0.375 % (w/v) TBA-15% (w/v) TCA-0.25N HCl reagent and incubated in boiling water bath for 30 minutes and centrifuged to obtain clear supernatant. Optical density (OD) was measured at 534 nm using UV VIS spectrophotometer (Thermo Scientific, USA) and results were expressed in (nmoles/gm Hb) nmols of MDA per gram of hemoglobin.

3.11.4 Protein Carbonyl (PCO):

Erythrocytic protein carbonyls (PCO) was measured according to the procedure of Levine et al., (1990). 0.2 ml hemolysate samples in PBS were mixed with 4.0 ml of 10 mM 2,4-dinitrophenylhydrazine (DNPH) prepared in 2 M HCl. The reaction mixture was incubated for 1 hour in the dark at 37 °C. After incubation, 20% TCA (w/v) was added and the mixture left in ice for 10 min. The clear supernatant was carefully aspirated and discarded. The protein pellets were washed three times with ethanol: ethyl acetate (1:1, v/v) solution to remove unreacted DNPH and lipid remnants. Finally protein pellets were dissolved in 6 M guanidine hydrochloride and incubated for 10 min at 37 °C. The insoluble materials were removed by centrifugation. The carbonyl content was determined by taking the spectra of the supernatant at 370 nm, using the molar extinction coefficient of DNPH, e=22000 M−1 cm−1 and result was expressed in (n mole/ g Hb or protein).

3.12 Assessment of Antioxidant enzymes:

3.12.1 Superoxide Dismutase activity (CuZn-SOD):

The activity of superoxide dismutase (SOD) was determined by the Marklund and Marklund (1974) with slight modifications. 50 µl of hemolysate was incubated with 0.05 M Tris succinate buffer (pH 8.5) at 37°C and reaction started by adding 0.1 ml of 20mM pyrogallol. The increase in absorbance (OD) was recorded at 420 nm for 3 min. The activity of SOD was expressed as (units/mg Hb) units per milligram hemoglobin.

3.12.2 Catalase (CAT):

The activity of Catalase can be measured by the method of Sinha et al., (1972). Mix Tris HCL (1M), EDTA (pH 8.0, 5mM, 50 µl), H_2O_2 (10 Mm, 900µl) and deionized water (30 µl). The decrease in absorbance was recorded at 240nm. Incubate the reaction mixture mixture at 37°C for 10 min. Catalase is expressed as unit per gram of hemoglobin (unit/g Hb or protein).

3.12.3 Glutathione Peroxidase (GPx) activity:

The activity of GPx was measured by method described by Rotruck et al., (1973). 0.02 ml of plasma was added to reaction mixture containing 500 µl of 0.02% GSH, 100 µl of 10 mM NaN_3, 100 µl of 10mM H_2O_2, 380 µl of distilled water and 400 µl of 0.1 M Tris-Cl buffer (pH 7.4). The reaction mixture was incubated at 37 °C for 15 minutes. Then, 0.3 ml of 10% TCA was added to stop the reaction and the tubes were centrifuged to obtain clear supernatant. To this supernatant, 2 ml of 0.3 M Na_2HPO_4 and 0.1ml of Ellman's reagent (19.5 g 5, 5'-dithiobisnitrobenzoic acid (DTNB) in 100ml 0.1% sodium citrate) was added. Standard curve for GSH was obtained simultaneously and absorbance of standard and test samples was read at 412 nm. The activity of GPx was expressed as µmol of GSH consumed/min/ml of plasma.

3.13. Total Antioxidant Activity (TAC) indexed as FRAP:

(Ferric Reducing Ability of Plasma)

The ferric reducing antioxidant power (FRAP) was estimated by the method of Benzie and Strain et al., (1996). 0.04 ml plasma was added to 2 ml of reaction mixture containing acetate buffer (pH 3.6, 10mM); 2, 4, 6-tripyridyl-s-triazine (TPTZ) in HCl (40 mM) and $FeCl_3.6H_2O$ (20 mM). Absorbance was measured against working FRAP at 593 nm through time scanning at 30 second intervals for 4 minutes. Increase in absorbance per minute was calculated for test plasma. The standard curve for 40 - 400µl $FeSO_4$ was also obtained. Quantification was done by regression analysis and the FRAP values were reported as µmol Fe (II)/ml of the plasma.

3.14. Measurement of Inflammatory Markers:

Inflammatory markers Human CRP was estimated by Automated Bioanalyzer kits (Accurax Biomedical) and Human TNF-α and IL-6 were estimated by ELISA kits (Elabscience) and the assay was performed according to the manufacturer's protocol.

3.14.1. Interleukin 6 (IL-6):

This ELISA kit uses the Sandwich-ELISA principle. The micro ELISA plate provided in this kit has been pre-coated with an antibody specific to Human IL-6. Standards or samples are added to the micro ELISA plate wells and combined with the specific antibody. Then a biotinylated detection antibody specific for Human IL-6 and Avidin-Horseradish Peroxidase (HRP) conjugate are added successively to each micro plate well and incubated. Free components are washed away. The substrate solution is added to each well. Only those wells that contain Human IL-6, biotinylated detection antibody and Avidin-HRP conjugate will appear blue in color. The enzyme-substrate reaction is terminated by the addition of stop solution and the color turns yellow. The optical density (OD) is measured spectrophotometrically at a wavelength of 450 nm ± 2 nm. The cytokine concentration was calculated using standard curve prepared by standard IL-6 (figure 3.3) and expressed as pg/ml.

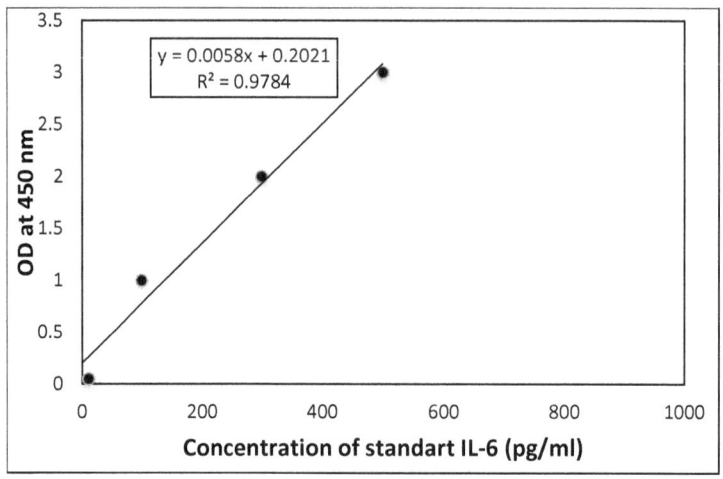

Figure 3.3. Standard Curve for IL-6

3.14.2. Tumor Necrosis Factor alpha (TNF-α):

The Human TNF α solid-phase sandwich ELISA (enzyme-linked immunosorbent assay) is designed to measure the amount of the target bound between a matched antibody pair. A target-specific antibody has been pre-coated in the wells of the supplied microplate. Samples, standards, or controls are then added into these wells and bind to the immobilized (capture) antibody. Then a biotinylated detection antibody specific for Human TNF-α and Avidin-Horseradish Peroxidase (HRP) conjugate are added successively to each micro plate well and incubated. The substrate solution is added to each well. Only those wells that contain Human TNF-α, biotinylated detection antibody and Avidin-HRP conjugate will appear blue in color. The enzyme-substrate reaction is terminated by the addition of stop solution and the color turns yellow. The optical density (OD) is measured spectrophotometrically at a wavelength of 450 nm ± 2 nm. The OD value is proportional to the concentration of Human TNF-α and expressed as pg/ml.

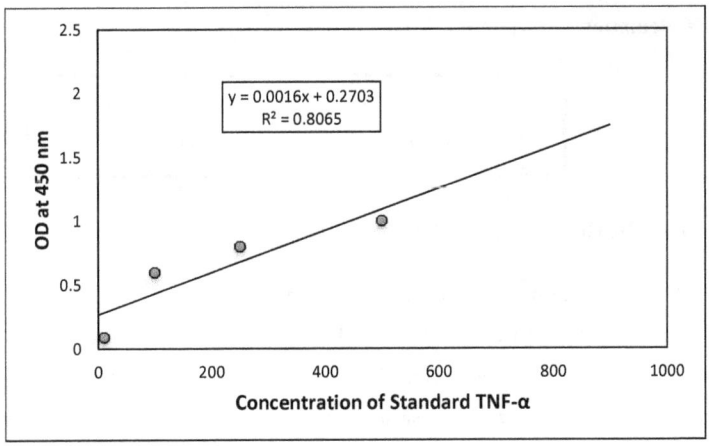

Figure 3. 4. Standard Curve for TNF –α

3.14.3. C- Reactive Protein (CRP):

High sensitivity C-Reactive Protein (hs-CRP) was determined by using Automated Analyzer method. Infinite Turbilatex CRP contain latex particle coated with specific anti-human CRP which reacts with CRP in the sample resulting in the agglutination.Agglutination causes changes in absorbance measured at 540nm(530-540 nm) and is proportional to the concentration of CRP in the sample. The reagent kit should be stored at 2 -8 °C and is stable till the expiry date indicated on the label. After collection of blood, serum were isolated, 5 µl of serum were mixed in working solution provided in standard clinical kits, and absorbance were taken. According to manual protocol a hs-CRP level of less than <1.0 mg/ml is considered to a low level, 1.0 to 2.0 mg/mL considered as intermediate level and greater then >2.5 mg/mL an elevated high risk.

Calculation

> Factor = Conc. of Calibrator / (A2-A1) Calibrator
>
> CRP mg/ml = (A2-A1)Sample × Factor

3.15. Statistical Analysis:

Statistical analysis was performed using Microsoft, Excel 2013, Prism Graph Pad 5 and JASP 0.8 software, Sigma Plot 10. All the results are presented as (mean±SD) mean ± standard deviation. The statistical significance of intergroup differences were assessed using one way analysis of variance (ANOVA), followed by post hoc Tukey's HSD test for parametric data sets and Kruskal Wallis test followed by Dunn's multiple comparisons for non parametric data sets to assess all pair wise differences. Pearson correlation coefficients were obtained to see relationship between different variables. Unless stated otherwise, all values at 95% confidence with $p<0.05$ were considered statistically significant. Receiver operating characteristic (ROC) curve and area under ROC curve (AUC) were calculated to find out odds ratio of OS markers by using sensitivity and specificity.

RESULTS AND DISCUSSION

Chapter 4.1: Section (A): To compare metabolically healthy (MH) non obese controls, overweight and obese respondents with regard to markers of NCEP ATP III MetS risk factors, oxidative stress, redox balance and inflammation.

The baseline characteristics of the study population, presented in Table 4.1.1,confirms that all groups, namely MHO, MHOw and MHNO based on their BMI are matched for gender, age and height, and are assigned to the MHOw and MHO groups based on their BMI.

Table 4.1.1: General characteristics of metabolically healthy non obese control (MHNO), metabolically healthy overweight (MHOw) and metabolically healthy obese (MHO).

Demographic Data	MHNO	MHOw	MHO
N	100	147	102
Male/Female	55/45	74/73	59/43
Age (year)	53.9±10.2	52.8±13.2	55.3±13.8
Height (cm)	160±7.8	158.7±6.3	159.6±6.5
Weight (kg)	59.7±7.2	66.4±6.6	82.8±6.4
BMI (kg/m^2)	22.8±1.5	26.9±1	32.6±1.3

All values are presented as mean ±SD.

NCEP ATP III diagnostic criteria [NCEP ATP, 2010] for metabolic syndrome (Met S) and other clinical biochemical measures, to define metabolic health (MH) in MHNO, MHOw and MHO obesity phenotypes are presented in Table 4.1.2.

Table 4.1.2: NCEP ATP III diagnostic criteria for Met S and other clinical biochemical measures, to describe MHNO, MHOw and MHO phenotypes.

Met S Risk Factors	Cut off Range	MHNO	MHOw	MHO	P value
NCEP ATP III Diagnostic Criteria For Met S					
Waist circumference	Men :≥90 cm Women :≥80 cm	75.4±8	85.6±9.7	101±11.9	<0.0001***
Fasting Blood Glucose	≥100 mg/dl	86.9±9.1	93.3±5.5	102.5±9.3	<0.0001***
Triglyceride	≥150 mg/dl	130±18.8	131.5±8.6	152.7±12.3	<0.0001***
HDL-Cholesterol	Men :≤ 40 mg/dl Women :≤ 50 mg/dl	54.3±7.1	53.1±5	49±6.5	<0.0001***
Blood Pressure	Systolic ≥130 mmHg	115±5.2	119.9±4.9	122.5±4.9	<0.0001***
	Diastolic >85 mmHg	75.8±7.2	79.2±4.2	80.9±4.8	<0.0001***
Other related biochemical measures					
Total Cholesterol	150- 250 mg/dl	176.7±10.8	181.7±10.3	200.2±14	<0.0001***
Low density lipoprotein-C	≤150 mg/dl	96.4±12.1	103.9±12.6	120.6±16.9	<0.0001***
Very low density Lipoprotein	5 - 40 mg/dl	30±10	28.5±10.9	20.8±3.1	<0.0001***

All values are presented as mean ±SD.

As dictated by the inclusion criteria, it was confirmed that all the metabolic syndrome diagnostic measures and other related biochemical measures do not fall outside the reference range as stated in the NCEP ATP III norms, except for waist circumference, as expected because screening was done on the basis of overweight/obesity. However, one way ANOVA confirmed that there was statistically significant difference among the groups at p< 0.05 for all risk factors, with the MHO showing more aberration than the MHOw, while, as expected the MHNO had the healthiest metabolic profile. Since one way ANOVA does not tell which pairs of groups are different from each other, Tukey's post hoc HSD test was performed.

Table 4.1.3: Results from Tukey's test for all parameters to assess pairwise significance between groups of metabolically healthy phenotypes.

	WC	BGF	TG	HDL	SBP	TC	LDL	VLDL	DBP
MHNO vs MHOw	***	***	ns	ns	**	**	*	ns	**
MHNO vs MHO	***	***	***	***	***	***	***	***	***
MHOw vs MHO	***	***	***	***	***	***	***	***	*

Data were processed for analysis for one way ANOVA followed by Tukey's test. One, two and three asterisks signify statistical significance at $p \leq 0.05$, $p \leq 0.005$ and $p \leq 0.0005$ respectively.

As seen from Table 4.1.3, it was found that MHOW did not differ significantly from MHNO with regard to triglycerides, HDL and VLDL, but their waist circumference, blood glucose fasting, and LDL were significantly higher. On the other hand, MHO vs MHNO, as well as MHO vs MHOw differed from each other with regard to all parameters.

Figure 4.1.1 represents the relative per cent difference of biochemical parameters between MHNO and MHOw, MHNO and MHO, and MHOw and MHO. Interestingly, the difference between MHOw and MHNO for all parameters except SBP and DBP, was minimum of all pairs studied, and was maximum for comparison between MHO and MHNO confirming the greater impact of obesity (BMI>30) than of overweight (BMI 25-30) on all parameters under study, even in metabolically healthy groups.

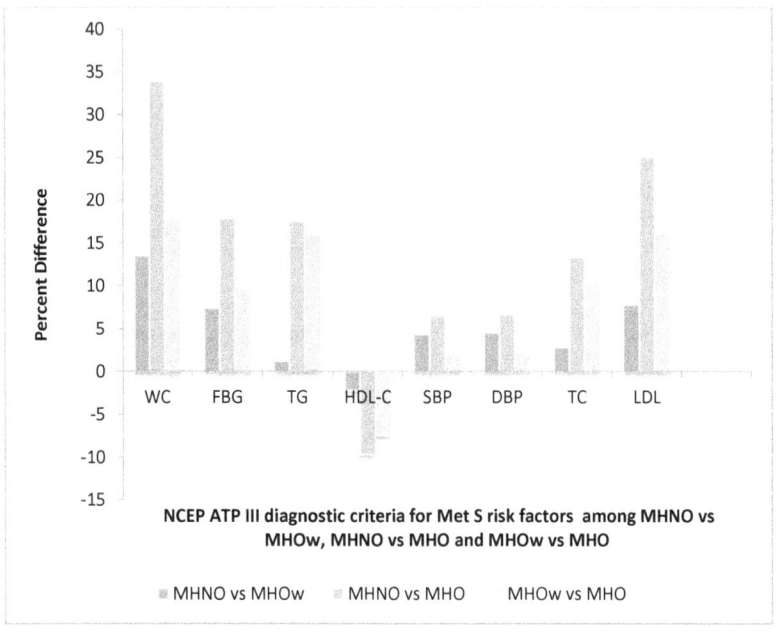

Figure 4.1.1: Relative per cent difference of NCEP ATP III diagnostic criteria for Met S, and related biochemical parameters between MHNO and MHOw, MHNO and MHO, and MHOw and MHO.

Abbreviation : WC: waist circumference, BGF: Blood glucose fasting, TG: triglycerides, HDL : High density lipoprotein, SBP: systolic blood pressure, TC: Total cholesterol, LDL :Low density lipoprotein.

Plasma/serum OS markers serum hydroxyl radical ($^\bullet$OH), plasma fluorescent oxidation products (FLOP), GPx, FRAP, erythrocytic oxidative stress markers: MDA, PCO, CuZn SOD, catalase and circulating (serum) inflammatory markers: C-reactive protein (CRP), tumor necrosis factor alpha (TNF $-\alpha$), interleukin 6 (IL- 6) were assessed in the three groups and results are presented in Table 4.1.4.

Table 4.1.4. Erythrocytic/plasma oxidative stress, antioxidant and inflammatory markers in MHNO, MHOW and MHO respondents.

Biochemical Markers	MHNO	MHOw	MHO	P value
Oxidative stress markers				
OH Radicals (µmol/L) (N=57+58+57)	256±32	294±54	413±60	<0.0001***
Fluorescent Oxidation Products (FI§/ml) (N=57+58+57)	169±19	176±31	193±39	0.0002***
MDA (nmoles/g Hb)	0.85±0.4	1.74±1	3.47±1	<0.0001***
PCO (nmole/g Hb)	0.45±0.1	0.89±0.6	2.55±0.8	<0.0001***
Antioxidant Markers				
CuZn SOD (unit /g Hb)	4±1.7	3.96±1.7	2.84±1	<0.0001***
CAT (unit/g Hb)	3.0±0.9	2.70±1	2.29±0.6	<0.0001***
GPX (nmole/min/mg plasma protein)	5.2±2	4.7±1.5	4.31±1.8	0.0008***
FRAP (µmole/ml of plasma)	4.3±1.5	4.05±1.5	2.97±0.9	<0.0001***
Inflammatory Markers				
CRP (mg/ml)	1.05±0.6	2±0.9	3±0.8$	<0.0001***
TNF–α (pg/ml) (N=36+31+35)	35.5±10	43.9±15	95.02±32	<0.0001***
IL 6 (pg/ml) (36+24+31)	6.3±1.6	10.5±1.2	16.7±6.7	<0.0001***

All the values are expressed as mean±SD. (•OH: Hydroxyl Radical, FLOP: Fluorescent Oxidation Products, MDA: Malondialdehyde, PCO: Protein carbonyl, SOD: Superoxide dismutase, FRAP: Ferric reducing ability of plasma, GPX: Glutathione Peroxidase, CAT: Catalase, CRP: C reactive protein, TNF–α: Tumor necrosis factor alpha, IL 6: Interleukin 6.)

One way ANOVA showed highly significant difference (p<0.0001) with regard to all parameters under study. A closer look at the data indicated that the difference between groups were not all significantly different from each other. Hence, Tukey's post hoc HSD test was performed and results were presented in Table 4.1.5.

Table 4.1.5: Post Hoc analysis using Tukeys test to assess comparisons between groups.

	OH Radicals	FLOP	MDA	PCO	CuZn SOD	CAT	GPx	FRAP	CRP	TNF–α	IL 6
MHNO vs MHOW	**	ns	***	***	ns	*	*	ns	***	***	***
MHNO vs MHO	***	**	***	***	***	***	***	***	***	***	***
MHOw vs MHO	***	*	***	***	***	**	ns	***	***	***	***

Data were processed for analysis for one way ANOVA followed by Tukeys test or Kruskal Wallis test followed by Dunns multiple comparison test at p<0.05.

Post hoc analysis revealed that differences between MHNO and MHOw were not significant with regard to FLOP antioxidant marker, CuZn SOD and total antioxidant capacity marker FRAP, and only marginally different with regard to catalase, GPx while lipid peroxidation marker MDA and protein carbonylation markers PCO showed significant difference. All markers were different in MHO group when compared with MHNO as well as when compared with MHOW. Inflammatory markers CRP, TNF alpha, and IL- 6 were significantly (p<0.0001) different from each other, as indicated by one-way ANOVA as well as by post hoc tests, comparing all pairs of groups, that is MHNO, with MHOw and with MHO, and MHOw with MHO.

When the results of OS markers were presented graphically Fig 4.2.2 (a), (b), (c), which represent the relative percent difference, it was again confirmed that differences with regard to all parameters, namely, serum hydroxyl radicals (•OH), plasma fluorescent oxidation products (FLOP), malondialdehyde (MDA) and protein carbonyl (PCO), CuZn-Superoxide dismutase (CuZn-SOD), glutathione peroxidase (GPx), catalase (CAT) and ferric reducing ability of plasma (FRAP), and C-reactive protein (CRP), tumor necrosis factor alpha (TNF $-\alpha$), interleukin 6 (IL- 6) were minimum between MHNO and MHOw groups, and maximum between MHO vs MHNO.

Relative per cent difference of biochemical parameters followed the sequence: between MHNO and MHO > between MHOw and MHO> between MHNO and MHOw. The differences between the normal weight healthy controls and their overweight counterparts was minimum with regard to most parameters studied.

Figure 4.1.2 (a)

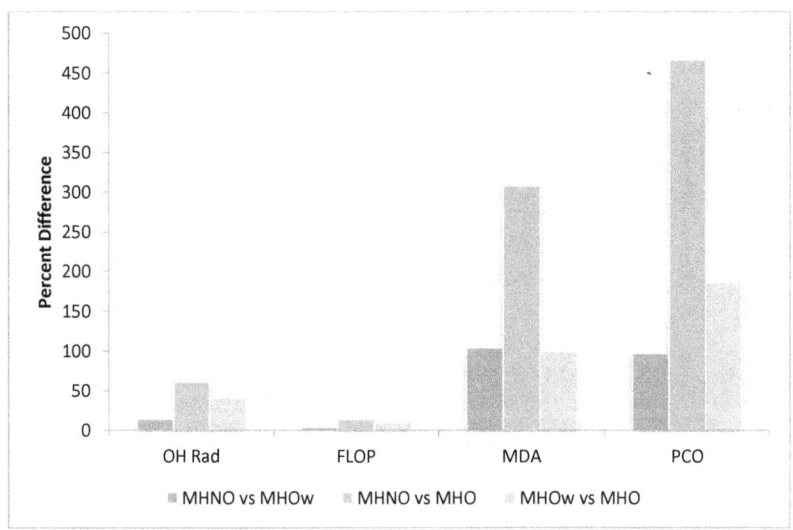

Figure 4.1.2(b) Figure 4.1.2 (c)

Results and Discussioun

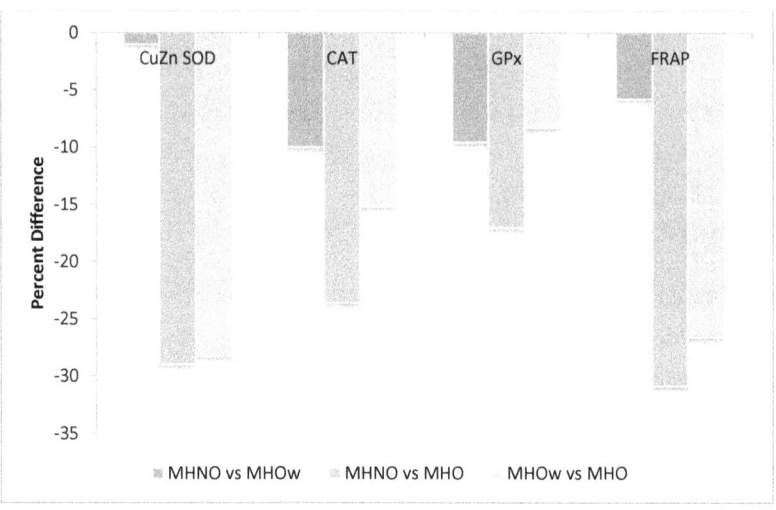

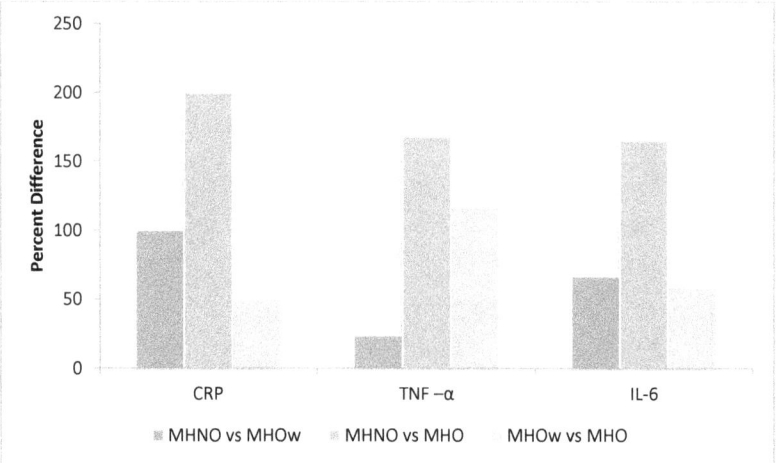

Figure 4.1.2: Relative per cent difference of biochemical parameters between MHNO and MHOw, MHNO and MHO and MHOw and MHO, with regard to (a) serum hydroxyl radicals (•OH), plasma fluorescent oxidation products (FLOP), malondialdehyde (MDA) and protein carbonyl (PCO), (b) CuZn Superoxide dismutase (CuZn SOD), glutathione peroxidase (GPx), catalase (CAT) and ferric reducing ability of plasma (FRAP), and (c) C reactive protein (CRP), tumor necrosis factor alpha (TNF –α), interleukin 6 (IL- 6).

Since the groups were categorized based on their BMI, relationship of selected OS markers, •OH Radicals, FLOP, and inflammatory markers, CRP, IL6 and TNF-α were assessed by calculating Pearson's correlation coefficients (Table 4.1.6).

Table 4.1.6: Pearson's correlation coefficients to assess relationships of BMI with OS, antioxidant markers and inflammatory for MHNO, MHO$_W$ and MHO.

		•OH Rad	FLOP	MDA	PCO	SOD	CAT	GPx	FRAP	CRP	TNF	IL6
BMI	MHNO	0.048	0.016	-0.130	-0.115	-0.234*	-0.118	-0.106	-0.134	0.07	-0.166	0.013
	MHOW	0.463*	0.368*	0.346*	0.288*	-0.289*	-0.154	-0.188	-0.271*	0.211	0.184	0.311*
	MHO	0.585*	0.618*	0.623*	0.535*	-0.369*	-0.254*	-0.345*	-0.341*	0.324*	0.599*	0.630*

Values marked with asterisk are statistically significant at $p \leq 0.05$.

All OS and inflammatory markers increased as severity of obesity, as measured by BMI increased, but MHNO did not show this pattern, as expected. BMI in MHO group showed strong positive correlation with all OS and inflammatory markers but antioxidant markers showed negative correlation with BMI while Controls (MHNO) did not show any significant pattern. The above results depict that as BMI increases, oxidative stress and inflammation both increase. These patterns indicate that the mechanism that causes the obesity related health consequences comprise reduction in antioxidant enzymes, CuZn SOD, CAT and GPx, leading to increase in OS markers OH, FLOP, MDA and PCO. Increasing BMI also resulted in increase in inflammatory markers CRP, IL6 and TNF- α. The correlations between OS, inflammatory and antioxidant markers versus BMI were presented in Fig. 4.1.3, to show the remarkably different patterns between MHNO and MHO respondents.

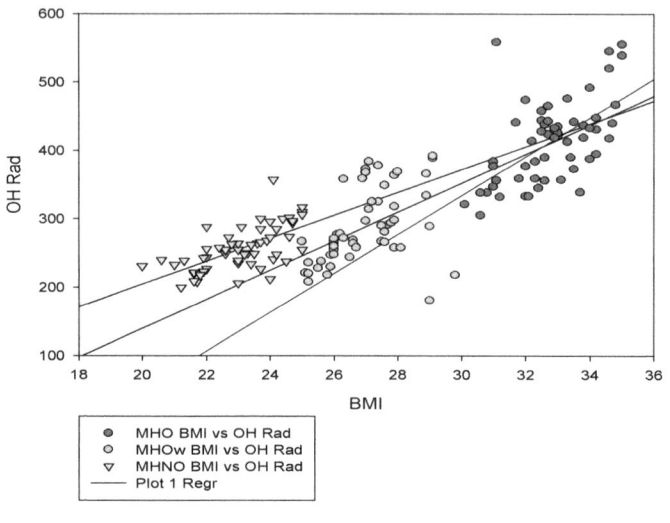

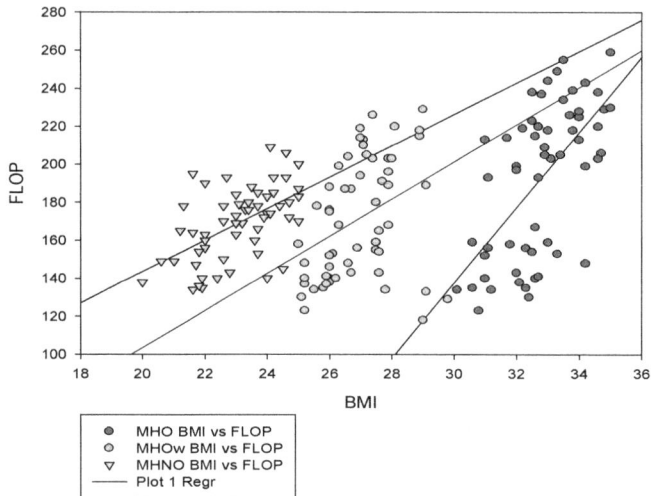

(c) MDA vs BMI **(d).** PCO vs BMI

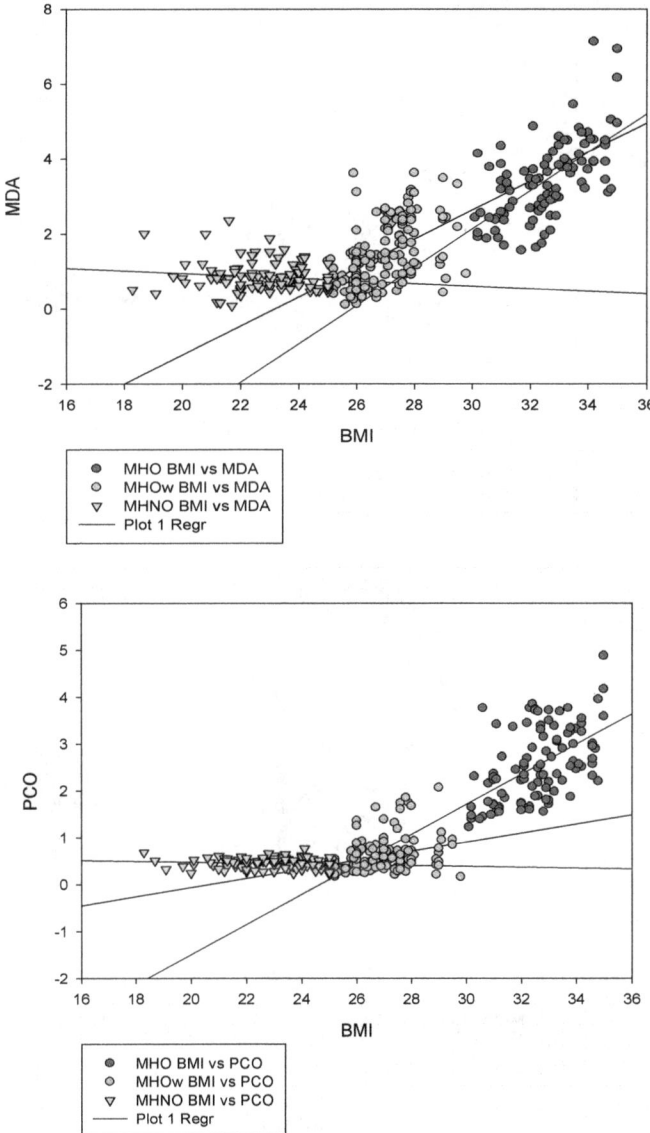

(e). CuZn SOD vs BMI **(f).** CAT vs BMI

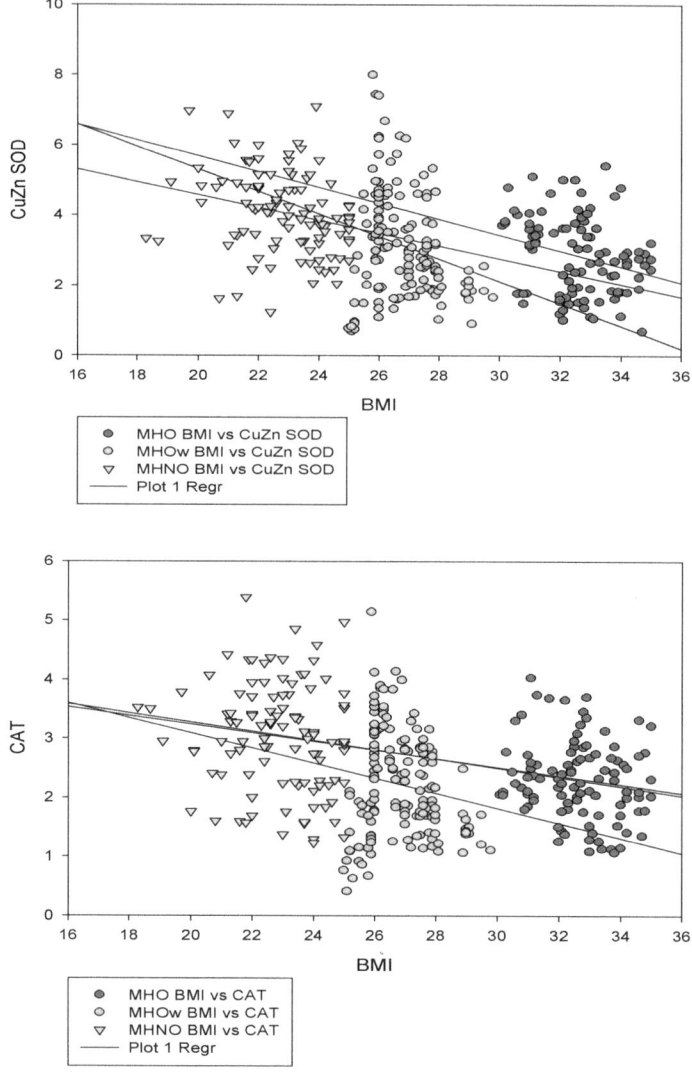

(g). GPx vs BMI **(h).** FRAP vs BMI

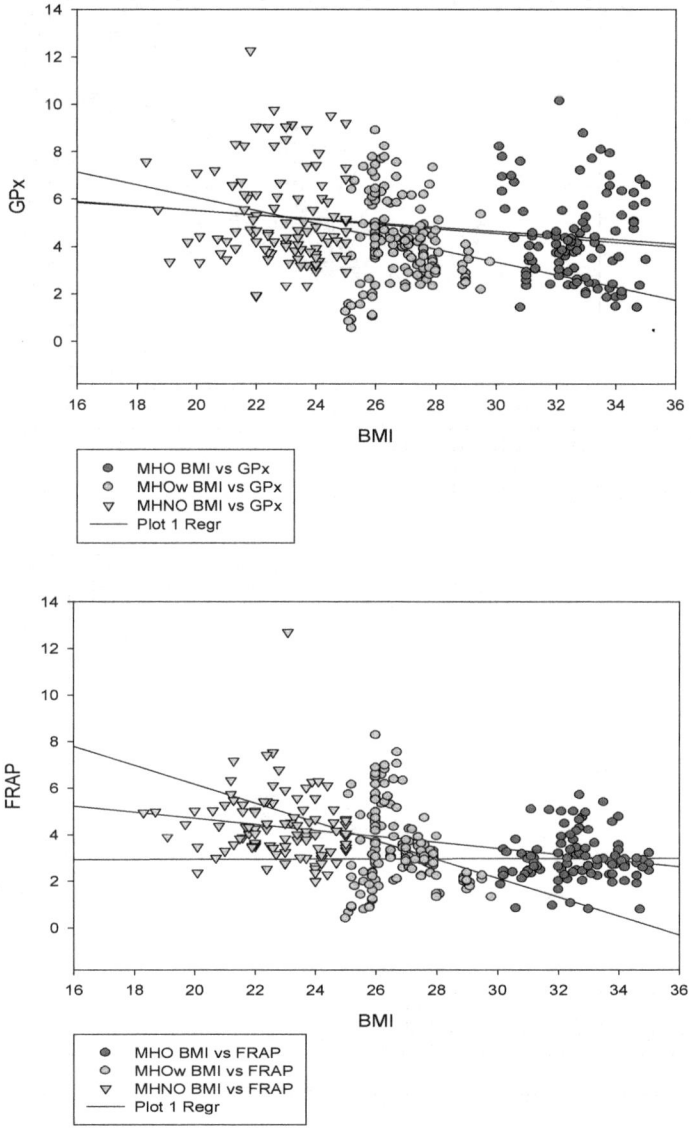

(i). CRP vs BMI **(j).** TNF alpha vs BMI

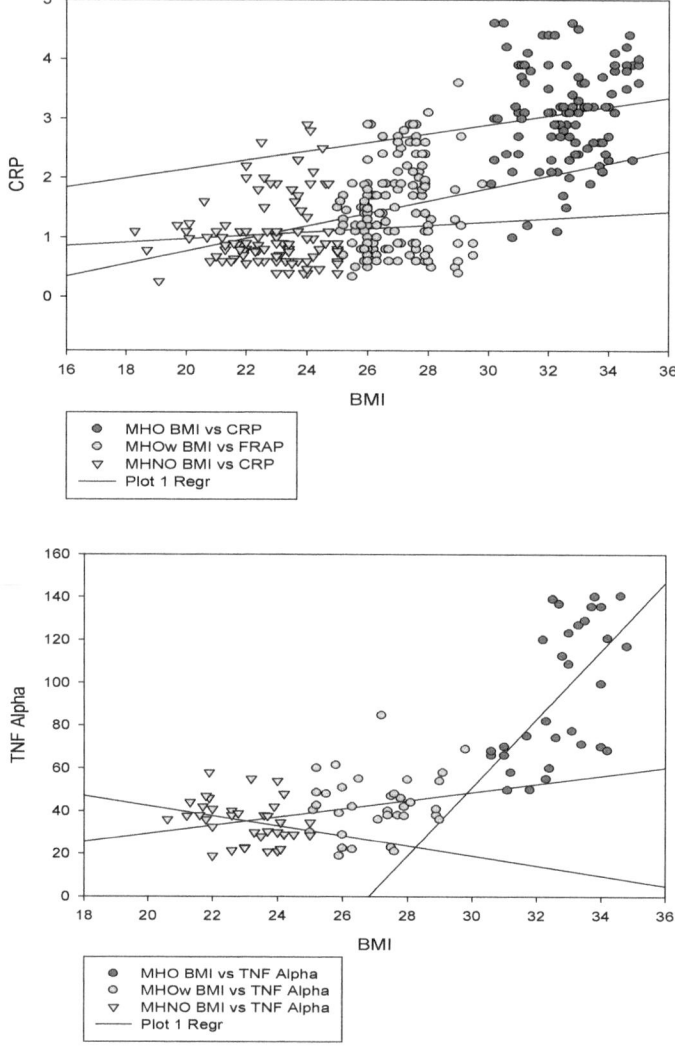

(k). IL 6 vs BMI

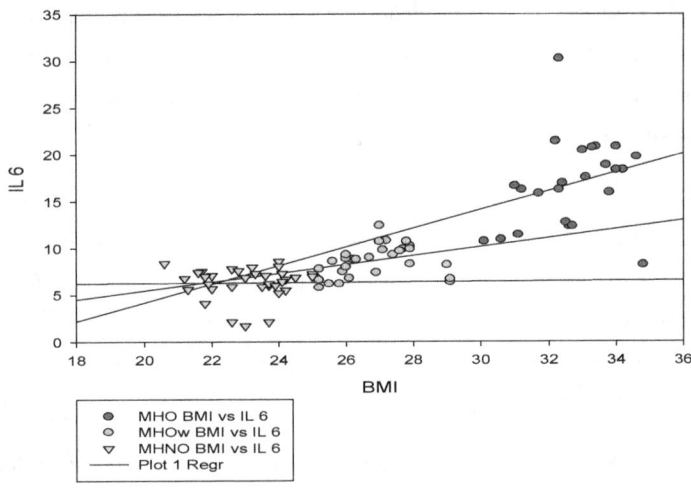

Fig 4.1.3 (a) OH Rad vs BMI (b). FLOP vs BMI

Figure 4.1.3. Correlation graphs for (a) OH Rad vs BMI (b) FLOP vs BMI (c) MDA vs BMI, (d) PCO vs BMI, (e) CuZn SOD vs BMI, (f) CAT vs BMI, (g) GPx vs BMI, (h) FRAP vs BMI, (i) CRP vs BMI, (j) TNF alpha vs BMI (k) IL 6 vs BMI between MHNO and MHO respondents.

Chapter 4.1. Section (B): Comparison of BMI classification guidelines with regard to NCEP ATP III Met S risk factors, oxidative stress and inflammatory markers among metabolically healthy (MH) non obese controls, overweight and obese respondents.

The currently most accepted categorization of obesity and overweight is body mass index (BMI), which is used within each population to identify the proportion of people with a high risk of an undesirable health state that warrants a public health or clinical intervention. WHO categorizes those with BMI≤25 kg/m^2 as non-obese; 25-30 kg/m^2 as overweight, and BMI>30 kg/m^2 as obese. However, there has been a debate on whether ethnic-specific cut-off points for BMI for Asians are required in the light of scientific evidence that Asian populations have different associations between BMI, percentage of body fat, and health risks than European populations. The Indian Consensus Group (for Asian Indians residing in India has per published definitive guidelines recommending revised guidelines for Asians, particularly Indians, to classify a BMI of ≥ 23 kg/m^2 and ≥ 25 kg/m^2 as overweight and obese. Thus the non-obese group according to the WHO criteria is divided into two groups.

To assess the logic of this division, we have regrouped the MHNO group (BMI 18-25) of Section A into two groups of the Asian classification, MHNO$_{Asian}$ and MHOw$_{Asian}$ and compared them with each other and with the MHNO$_{WHO}$ as described in Table 4.1.B1. The three groups were compared in pairs using the Tukey's post hoc test as represented in Table 4.1.B2.

Table 4.1.B1: NCEP ATP III diagnostic criteria for MetS, other biochemical measures, OS markers and inflammatory markers defined by WHO and revised consensus guidelines for India.

Met S risk factors	MHNOWHO (BMI:18-24.9)	MHNOAsian (BMI: 18-22.9)	MHOwAsian (BMI: 23-24.9)
NCEP ATP III risk factors for MetS			
Waist circumference	75.4±8	72.2±8.5	76.3±6.5
Fasting Plasma Glucose	86.9±9.1	83.5±7	85.4±8.6
Triglyceride	130±18.8	126.8±17.3	128.5±18.8
HDL-Cholesterol	54.3±7.1	54.4±6.9	54±7.3
Systolic Blood Pressure	115±5.2	115.1±5.3	116.3±5.3
Diastolic Blood Pressure	75.8±7.2	75.7±7.1	76.2±6.4
Total Cholesterol	176.7±10.8	174.9±9.9	177.8±10.3
Low density lipoprotein-C	96.4±12.1	95.2±12.3	98.1±12.4
Very low density Lipoprotein-C	30±10	29.8±10.3	29.5±9.6
Oxidative Stress Markers			

Serum OH Radicals (μmol/L)	256±32	237±22	268±32
Serum FLOP (FI§/ml)	169±19	157±18	162±15
Erythrocytic MDA (nmoles/g Hb)	0.85±0.4	0.8±0.4	0.8±0.3
Erythrocytic PCO (nmole/g Hb)	0.45±0.1	0.4±0.1	0.4±0.1
CuZn-SOD (unit /g Hb)	4±1.7	3.9±1.3	3.9±1.2
CAT (unit/g Hb)	3.0±0.9	2.9±0.9	2.9±1.9
Plasma GPX (nmole/min/mg plasmaprotein)	5.2±2	4.9±1.9	4.9±1.9
FRAP (μmole/ml of plasma)	4.3±1.5	4.3±1.3	4.1±1.7
Inflammatory Markers			
CRP (mg/ml)	1.05±0.6	1±0.5	1±0.5
TNF–α (pg/ml)	35.5±10	32.6±10.3	37.6±8.2
IL 6 (pg/ml)	6.3±1.6	6.1±1.9	6.2±1.5

All the values are expressed as mean±SD. *(•OH: Hydroxyl Radical, FLOP: Fluorescent Oxidation Products, MDA: Malondialdehyde, PCO: Protein carbonyl, SOD: Superoxide dismutase, FRAP: Ferric reducing ability of plasma, GPX: Glutathione Peroxidase, CAT: Catalase, CRP: C reactive protein, TNF–α: Tumor necrosis factor alpha, IL 6: Interleukin 6).*

NCEP ATP III risk factors for MetS, OS and inflammatory markers to compare various pairs of metabolically healthy respondents, distributed according to BMI cut offs stratified by WHO and revised consensus guidelines for India. The biochemical parameters including triglyceride, HDL-cholesterol, systolic and diastolic blood pressure, LDL and VLDL did not show significant difference from each other group. Similar results were also found for MDA, PCO, CuZn SOD, CAT, GPx and FRAP except OH radicals and FLOPs.

Table 4.1.B2: Post Hoc analysis using Tukeys' test to assess comparisons between groups.

Post hoc Analysis by Tukey's HSD Test			
	$MHNO_{WHO}$ vs $MHNO_{Asian}$	$MHNO_{WHO}$ vs $MHOw_{Asian}$	$MHNO_{Asian}$ vs $MHOw_{Asian}$
WC	*	ns	**
FPG	*	ns	ns
TG	ns	ns	ns
HDL-C	ns	ns	ns
SBP	ns	ns	ns
DBP	ns	ns	ns
TC	ns	ns	ns
LDL-C	ns	ns	ns
VLDL	ns	ns	ns
OH Radicals	*	ns	**
FLOPs	*	ns	***
MDA	ns	ns	ns
PCO	ns	ns	ns
CuZn SOD	ns	ns	ns
CAT	ns	ns	ns
GPx	ns	ns	ns
FRAP	ns	ns	ns
CRP	ns	ns	ns
TNF –α	ns	ns	ns
IL 6	ns	ns	ns

Data were processed for analysis for one way ANOVA followed by Tukeys test or Kruskal Wallis test followed by Dunns multiple comparison test at p<0.05.

Tukeys post hoc test compared various groups in pairs. No significant difference was found between $MHNO_{WHO}$ vs $MHNO_{Asian}$, $MHNO_{WHO}$ vs $MHOw_{Asian}$ and $MHNO_{Asian}$ vs $MHOw_{Asian}$ groups with regard to any parameters including all NCEP-ATPIII risk factors, OS, antioxidant markers and inflammatory markers while OH radicals and

FLOP showed significant difference in MHNO$_{WHO}$ vs MHNO$_{Asian}$ and MHNO$_{Asian}$ vs MHOw$_{Asian}$.

Discussion

The present study was conducted on metabolically healthy respondents, who were categorized as a healthier phenotype [Goossens G H., 2017] because all risk factors for metabolic syndrome as approved by the NCEP ATP III criteria were within the prescribed cut off range. Within this phenotype, the effects of body mass index (BMI) on various blood parameters, namely NCEP ATP III prescribed MetS risk factors, oxidative stress indices and selected inflammatory markers were investigated.

As described earlier, the study was divided into two sections A and B, based on the norms used to categorize obesity using BMI.

In Section A, the respondents are categorized according to the widely accepted WHO norms (BMI$\leq$25 kg/m^2; 25-30 kg/m^2, and BMI>30 kg/m^2 for MHNO, MNOw and MHO respectively), while in Section B, the Asian Guidelines were adopted which divided the MHNO group into two subgroups of BMI $\geq$ 23 kg/m^2 and $\geq$ 25 kg/m^2 as overweight and obese. Thus the non-obese group according to the WHO criteria is divided into two groups.

In Section A, within the NCEP-ATP permitted range, maximum percent difference was found for LDL, followed by fasting blood glucose (FBG) and triglyceride (TG) and reverse pattern was obtained for HDL as BMI increased from the MHNO, MHOW and MHO groups in that order. When the groups were reorganized in section B, no significant difference in any of NCEP ATP III risk factors except waist circumference (WC) and fasting plasma glucose (FPG), indicating that MHNO$_{Asian}$ and MHOw$_{Asian}$ belong to same group as recommended by WHO. Although the metabolically healthy phenotype has been so named because of its healthier metabolic profile, it has been suggested that they are on the way to becoming 'unhealthy' obese [Goossens G H., 2017] and the obese among these have been found to be at increased risk for (cardio) metabolic disease and type 2 diabetes [Hashimoto Y, Hamaguchi M,

Tanaka M et al., 2018] and may have other comorbidities. The data obtained does not indicate need for the modified Asian guidelines.

Metabolic diseases such as Diabetes mellitus, hypertension, dyslipidemia which can lead to cardiac disease are known to be associated with increased oxidative stress and disruptions in redox balance. Hence OS markers, namely, serum hydroxyl radicals and FLOP, MDA, PCO, antioxidant markers CuZn SOD, CAT, plasma GPx and total antioxidant activity in terms of FRAP were measured. Significant difference among groups was observed when assessed using one-way ANOVA. Tukeys' post hoc test was conducted to assess differences between pairs of groups. No significant difference was found between the MHNO and their MHO_W counterparts for any OS marker except MDA and PCO. The antioxidant enzymes, CuZn SOD, did not differ between the MHNO and MHO_W groups, while there was minimal difference between catalase and GPx. Consequently, overall antioxidant capacity indicator FRAP did not differ between the Controls and their overweight counterparts, leading to similar total antioxidant capacity. However, this pattern was not found in MHO phenotypes, where FRAP was significantly lowered, indicating the breakdown of redox homeostasis in MHO phenotypes due to significant reduction in antioxidant enzymes. This confirmed previous findings from various studies from our lab [Singh S, Dwivedi A, Kumar S et al., 2019], which have reported that increase in erythrocytic oxidative stress damage markers, malondialdehyde as well as protein carbonyls is generally accompanied by a decline in the erythrocytic antioxidant enzymes, super oxide dismutase and catalase, reflected in a decline in the FRAP value. Since, FRAP is an index of non-enzymatic total antioxidant capacity, it is suggested that the entire systemic milieu is interconnected and the overall homeostatic processes are linked. The normal weight Controls had the best homeostasis, which was sustained in the overweight group.

In Section B, the MHNO group is subdivided into two groups as recommended by the Asian Consensus Guidelines [Misra A., 2015] because Asians display a greater proportion of body fat for a given BMI than white Europeans [Rush EC, Goedecke JH, Jennings C et al., 2007] to assess whether ethnic-specific cut-off points for BMI for Asians are required in terms of oxidative stress and redox balance. Post hoc

Tukeys test revealed no significant difference for OS and antioxidant markers in MHNO$_{WHO}$ vs MHNO$_{Asian}$, MHNO$_{WHO}$ vs MHOw$_{Asian}$ and even in MHNO $_{Asian}$ vs MHOw$_{Asian}$ except a minor but significant difference between OH radicals and FLOP, indicating lack of support for the ethnic specific reorganization of Asian BMI criteria.

These findings were supported by the study of Kim et al. who compared metabolically healthy overweight (MHO) and metabolically unhealthy overweight (MUO) phenotypes matched for body mass index, lean body masses and total body fat percentages. They reported that plasma metabolomics revealed higher oxidative stress induced lipid peroxidation and protein carbonylation, which causes tissue damage in MUO as measured by higher levels of lipoprotein-associated phospholipase A$_2$(Lp-PLA$_2$), glycolic acid, 6-lysophosphatidylethanolamines (lysoPEs), and 12 lysophosphatidylcholines (lysoPCs) activity and higher levels of urinary 8-epi-prostaglandin F$_{2\alpha}$(8-epi-PGF$_{2\alpha}$) and oxidized low-density lipoprotein (ox-LDL) [Han Y, Kim M, JinYoo H et al., 2019]. In another comparative study to assess differences between metabolically healthy morbidly obese (MHMO) and metabolically unhealthy morbidly obese with MetS (MUHMO), no significant difference was found with regard to oxidative stress markers in terms of total oxidant status (TOS) and total antioxidant response (TAR) [Catoi AF., Pârvu AE, Andricut AD. et al., 2018].

The spectrofluorometer based oxidative stress markers ˙OH radicals and FLOP are highly sensitive. But they do not show significant difference between MHNO and MHOw groups. As stated earlier [Goossens G H., 2017] although MHO phenotypes are associated with healthier metabolic profile, it should not be regarded as a risk-free condition because these phenotypes have higher tendency for development of cardiometabolic diseases. Plasma FLOP is regarded as independent risk marker for prediction of cardiovascular diseases in epidemiological studies [Wu T, Rifai N, Willett WC et al., 2007], but has not been investigated to assess the differences in various grades of metabolically healthy obesity (MHO) hence the observed differences in ˙OH radicals and FLOP in different obesity grades in the present study assumes importance.

A study conducted on metabolically healthy obese postmenopausal women has revealed from metabolic profiling that lower concentration of hepatic circulating alanine transaminase (ALT) reflects lower liver fat content and lower hepatic insulin resistance [Messier V, Karelis AD, Robillard ME et al., 2011]. In another study, Wilkund et al [Wiklund P, Pekkala S, Autio R et al., 2014] reported that physically inactive overweight/obese women with metabolic syndrome and metabolically healthy overweight/obese women can be distinguished on the basis of metabolomics approach. They reported that branched-chain amino acids, orosomucoid and aromatic amino acids served as serum biomarkers to differentiate these two groups.

Inflammatory markers, CRP, TNF- α and IL-6 are known to be secreted by adipose tissue and are an index marker of obesity. They are also not found to be different between the MHNO and MHO$_W$ phenotype, and show a much higher value in the MHO phenotype. Further, all these parameters were significantly positively or negatively correlated to BMI, as expected. This indicates that as BMI increases, inflammation increases. It has been reported that level of inflammatory markers in different metabolically healthy obesity grades is highly dependent on adipose tissue distribution [Goossens G H., 2017]. Our findings suggest higher level of inflammatory markers in MHO phenotype. In a similar study conducted on Korean individuals, it was found that serum adipocytokines, TNF-α and adipocyte fatty acid binding protein (A-FABP) were lower in metabolically healthy obese and non-obese and significantly linked to metabolic unhealthiest in non-obese Korean individuals [Lee TH, Jeon WS, Han KJ et al., 2015]. Epidemiological evidence has demonstrated that normal adipose tissue function has been associated to healthier metabolic profile even in obese phenotypes [Bluher M., 2010]. TNF- α is multifunctional regulatory cytokine, secreted from macrophages of adipose tissue. The expression profiles of TNF- α changes the level of other proinflammatory adipocytokines and IL 6. In addition, it has been considered to be an important proinflammatory marker in development of obesity and its related comorbidities [Schmidt MI., Duncan BB., Sharrett AR. Et al., 1999]. Increased level of IL 6 is responsible for production of hs-CRP by liver as an important factor of the clinical inflammation in obesity. [Laaksonen DE., Niskanen L, Nyyssönen K et al., 2004].

Our results showed that there was little difference between the MHNO and MHO_W in the biochemical markers related to oxidative stress as well as inflammatory markers, but the impact of BMI in MHO group was significant on oxidative stress parameters as well as inflammatory markers. This raised questions on the healthier outcomes of the metabolically healthy phenotype. For example, it has been suggested that that this healthier metabolic profile may not translate into a lower risk for mortality [Primeau V, Coderre L, Karelis AD et al., 2011].

Mechanisms that could explain the favorable metabolic profile of MHO individuals are poorly understood, and may include differences in visceral fat accumulation, birth weight, adipose cell size and gene expression-encoding markers of adipose cell differentiation, which may favor the development of the MHO phenotype. The present study is part of the endeavor to make in depth study of the underlying cause-effect relationships. Collectively, a greater understanding of the MHO individual has important implications for therapeutic decision making, the characterization of subjects in research protocols and medical education. Lack of difference in inflammatory markers between metabolically healthy non-obese and their overweight counterparts may be because of the location where the excessive calories are stored. Location and function of adipose tissue are linked and determine metabolic health. Adipose tissue inflammation may be an adaptive response that enables safe storage of excess nutrients in adipose tissue, thereby protecting against metabolic and inflammatory perturbations and consequent comorbidities [Goossens G H., 2017]. For example, it has been demonstrated that in vivo IL-6 release from gluteofemoral adipose tissue was markedly lower than from the corresponding abdominal subcutaneous fat depot both in men and women [Pinnick KE, Nicholson G, Manolopoulos KN et al., 2014], suggesting that lower body fat may have a more beneficial inflammatory phenotype. These differences in disease risk are due to strikingly divergent functional properties of these adipose tissue depots, explaining.the difference seen in various metabolically healthy groups in the present study. Accumulation of adipose tissue in the upper body (abdominal region) is associated with the development of obesity-related comorbidities and even all-cause mortality.

Our findings of Section B suggest that there is no justification for subdividing the WHO prescribed Normal BMI range into two subgroups of Normal and overweight. In this connection, a study was designed to examine prevalence of the different metabolic phenotypes based on Asian Indian BMI cut offs and to distinguish between unhealthy and healthy metabolic profile belonging to different phenotypes of obesity [Bhansali S, Bhansali A, Dhawan V., 2017]. It was concluded that a healthy obese phenotype was associated with a better metabolic profile like lower blood glucose level, than observed in normal weight individuals with MetS, and increasing BMI had a significantly greater effect on estimates of liver fat and future CVD risk among those with MetS compared with participants without MetS.

We can conclude from this chapter that metabolic phenotyping of obese persons gives a perspective of the pathophysiology associated with obesity to identify the high risk subgroups that may help in optimization of prevention and management strategies to combat risk factors associated with the metabolic syndrome.

Chapter 4.2: To compare metabolically healthy non obese controls (MHNO), metabolically healthy overweight (MHOw) and metabolically healthy obese (MHO) respondents with regard to markers of NCEP ATP III Met S risk factors, oxidative stress, redox balance and inflammation in relation to age.

As seen from Chapter 4.1, no major differences were found when respondents are grouped by the more universally accepted WHO criteria for classification of respondents into normal, overweight and obese groups or by the less prevalent Asian Consensus Guidelines. Hence all further analysis was performed using the WHO criteria for BMI based classification.

As reported in Chapter 4.1, comparisons of various NCEP ATP III risk factors, oxidative stress markers between healthy normal weight controls and their overweight counterparts were found to be minimal but were more pronounced between MH overweight and MH obese groups. All metabolically healthy groups differed from each other with regard to inflammatory markers.

Since there is dearth of data on metabolically healthy overweight and obese persons many of the biochemical changes studied here can be expected to be age related. Hence, it was important to assess the impact of age on these parameters on the metabolically healthy respondents of various groups namely, normal weight controls, and their overweight and obese counterparts. Hence, chapter 4.2 was undertaken with the objective of comparing metabolically healthy non obese controls (MHNO), metabolically healthy overweight (MHOw) and metabolically healthy obese (MHO) respondents with regard to markers of oxidative stress, redox balance and inflammation in relation to age.

The respondents of three study groups MHNO, MHOw and MHO, aged 20-80 years were divided into three age groups, Young Adults (YA, 20-39 years), Middle-aged Adults (MA, 40-59 years), and Elderly (EA, 60 years). Table 4.2.1 represents the general characteristics of the study groups.

Table 4.2.1 General characteristics of the three age groups (20-39, 40-59 and ≥60) in metabolically healthy Control (MHNO), MH overweight (MHOw) and Obese (MHO) respondents

		Young adults (YA, 20-39 years)	Middle aged adults (MA, 40-59 years)	Elderly (EA, ≥60 years)	P value
Sample size n	MHNO	15	52	33	-
	MHOw	28	69	50	-
	MHO	14	50	38	-
Height (cm)	MHNO	160.6±9.2	159.1±7.5	161.4±7.3	-
	MHOw	157.7±6	158.7±5.7	159.3±7	-
	MHO	160.6±5	159.2±6.4	160±6.4	-
Weight (Kg)	MHNO	59.5±7	58.4±6.7	62.2±7.7	<0.0001***
	MHOw	63.1±4.7	66.3±6.3	67.9±7.4	0.008**
	MHO	81±6.9	81.6±6.2	85.3±5.9	0.003**
Body Mass Index (Kg/m2)	MHNO	22.1±1.7	22.7±1.5	23.4±1.5	0.019*
	MHOw	25.7±0.4	26.9±0.9	27.5±1	<0.0001***
	MHO	31.3±1.3	32.2±0.9	33.6±0.9	<0.0001***

All values are presented as mean ±SD

The impact of age on weight and BMI was assessed by One-way ANOVA and a statistically significant increase was observed in all groups as age increased.

The statistically significant positive correlation between age and body weight and between age and BMI in all metabolically healthy groups is confirmed and presented graphically in Fig 4.2.1.

Figure 4.2.1 (a) Age vs body weight   *Figure 4.2.1(b) Age vs BMI*

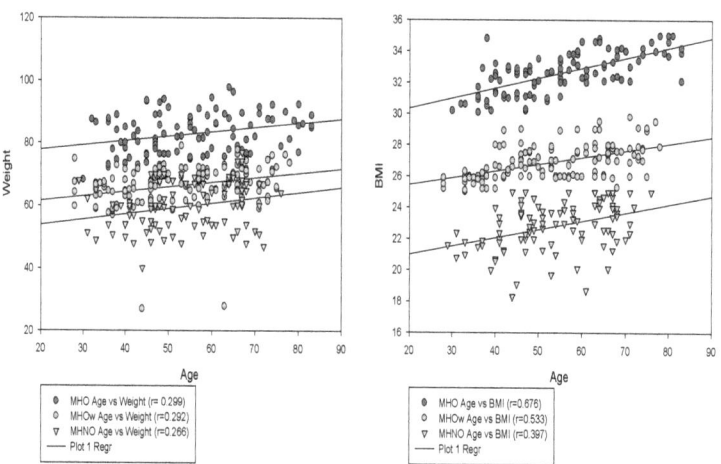

Fig 4.2.1. Relationship between age and (a) body weight (b) BMI in MHNO, MHOw and MHO respondents.

The Met S risk factors and other biochemical measures were analyzed in MHNO, MHOw and MHO respondents in three different age groups are presented in Table 4.2.2.

Table 4.2.2. Age- wise distribution of Met S risk factors and other biochemical measures in MHNO, MHOw and MHO group respondents.

		Young adults (YA, 20-39 years)	Middle aged adults (MA, 40-59 years)	Elderly (EA, ≥60 years)	ANOVA F value	ANOVA P value
NCEP :ATP III Diagnostic Criteria For Met S						
Waist Circumference Men:≥90cm Women :≥80 cm	MHNO	72.6±9.8	75.3±8.4	75.9±6.6	0.75	0.48
	MHOw	75.8±5.7	86.1±8.8	91.1±7.9	31.9	<0.0001** *
	MHO	94.2±12.3	99.8±11.5	104.6±11	4.68	0.011*
	P value	0.034**	<0.0001** *	<0.0001** *		
Fasting Plasma Glucose >100 mg/dl	MHNO	87.6±8.1	86.8±8.5	86.9±10.3	0.03	0.96
	MHOw	89.9±6.7	93.6±4.7	95±4.9	8.65	0.0003***
	MHO	101.1±9.8	103.5±9.2	102.8±10	0.35	0.70
	P value	<0.0001* **	<0.0001** *	<0.0001** *		
Triglycerides ≥150 mg/dl	MHNO	133±19.7	131.6±19.5	127.3±16.8	0.68	0.50
	MHOw	122.4±4.2	131.3±7.8	137.4±6.7	41.01	<0.0001** *
	MHO	153.3±12.7	151.7±12	152.9±12.7	0.14	0.87
	P value	<0.0001* **	<0.0001** *	<0.0001** *		
HDL-Cholesterol Men :≤ 40 mg/dl Women :≤ 50 mg/dl	MHNO	56.2±5.3	54±7.4	53.6±6.8	0.9	0.81
	MHOw	56.1±2.7	50.9±4.2	49±4	29.7	<0.0001** *
	MHO	51±4.8	50.9±5.4	45±7.1	9.2	0.0002***
	P value	0.0005** *	0.0048**	<0.0001** *		
Systolic Blood Pressure Systolic ≥130 mmHg	MHNO	115±4.4	114.8±5.4	115.7±5.3	0.32	0.72
	MHOw	118.8±5.9	120.9±4.3	119.1±5.1	2.88	0.05
	MHO	113.4±7.5	121.9±4.7	123 ±4.9	0.77	0.46
	P value	0.002**	<0.0001** *	<0.0001** *		
Other related biochemical measures						
Diastolic Blood Pressure Diastolic ≥80 mmHg	MHNO	74±5.6	75.8±7.1	77.1±7.9	0.80	0.45
	MHOw	80±3.1	78.3±4.7	79.7±3.7	2.5	0.08
	MHO	82.4±5.6	80±4	82±5.4	2.68	0.07
	P value	<0.0001* **	0.0006***	0.0016**		
	MHNO	176±12.3	177±9.6	175.5±12.3	0.23	0.79

Total Cholesterol 150-250 mg/dl	MHOw	170.4±4.3	182.1±9.5	187.7±8.5	37.2	0.001*
	MHO	195.1±5	199.9±14.2	202.3±15.3	1.41	0.25
	P value	<0.0001***	<0.0001**	<0.0001***		
Low Density Lipoprotein ≤150 mg/dl	MHNO	93.3±16.3	96.7±11.4	96.3±12.2	0.37	0.69
	MHOw	89.8±5.9	104.9±10.9	112.2±10.9	39.19	<0.0001**
	MHO	113.4±7.5	118.5±15.2	126±19.7	3.86	0.024*
	P value	<0.0001***	<0.0001**	<0.0001***		

		Tukey's Post hoc Test		
		YA vs. MA	YA vs. EA	MA vs. EA
WC	MHNO	ns	ns	ns
	MHOw	***	***	**
	MHO	ns	*	ns
FBG	MHNO	ns	ns	ns
	MHOw	**	***	ns
	MHO	ns	ns	ns
TG	MHNO	ns	ns	ns
	MHOw	***	***	***
	MHO	ns	ns	ns
HDL	MHNO	ns	ns	ns
	MHOw	***	***	*
	MHO	ns	*	***
SBP	MHNO	ns	ns	ns
	MHOw	ns	ns	ns
	MHO	ns	ns	ns
DBP	MHNO	ns	ns	ns
	MHOw	ns	ns	ns
	MHO	ns	ns	ns
TC	MHNO	ns	ns	ns
	MHOw	***	***	***
	MHO	ns	ns	ns
LDL	MHNO	ns	ns	ns
	MHOw	***	***	***
	MHO	ns	*	ns

All values are presented as mean ±SD. *Data were processed for analysis for one way ANOVA followed by Tukey's test. One, two and three asterisks signify statistical significance at p≤0.05, p≤0.005 and p≤0.0005 respectively.*

Cut-offs prescribed by NCEP-ATP III criteria: Waist circumference (WC): Men :≥90 cm, Women :≥80cm;Plasma fasting glucose (FPG): ≥100 mg/dl; Triglyceride (TG):

≥150 mg/dl, HDL Cholesterol (HDL-C): Men :≤ 40 mg/dl Women :≤ 50 mg/dl; blood pressure (BP): Systolic (SBP) ≥130 mmHg, Diastolic (DBP)>85 mmHg; total cholesterol (TC): 150- 250 mg/dl, low density lipoprotein (LDL-C): ≤150 mg/dl.

It can been seen from Table 4.2.2 that the mean values of NCEP ATP III criteria, namely waist circumference, fasting blood glucose, triglyceride, blood pressure as well as other related biochemical measures, namely total cholesterol, LDL-cholesterol and VLDL-cholesterol values fall in normal range, confirming metabolic health in all groups, MHNO, MHOw and MHO respondents. However, one way ANOVA confirmed that there was statistically significant difference in WC, FBG, TG, HDL-C, SBP, TC, and LDL, but not DBP with age in MHOw but not in MHNO and MHO groups. Since one way ANOVA does not tell which pairs of groups are different from each other, Tukey's post hoc HSD test was performed and this pattern was confirmed. A closer look at the values indicated that younger MHNO respondents began with a healthy profile which was retained as they aged, while the young MHO began with an unhealthy profile which did not worsen with age. MHNO group showed healthiest metabolic profile and MHO the unhealthiest, for all age groups but it did not worsen with age. On the other hand, the young MHOw showed a healthy profile which grew towards becoming unhealthy as they aged. One way ANOVA also found significant impact of BMI (that is grouping into MHNO, MHOw and MHO) for each age group for all NCEP ATP III risk factors and other related biochemical measures.

OS indices of the three age categories of MHNO, MHOw and MHO respondents were analyzed and findings are presented in Table 4.2.3, to investigate whether increasing age has a differential impact on body weight and redox status.

Table 4.2.3. Age- wise distribution of erythrocytic and plasma oxidative stress markers and antioxidant status of MHNO, MHOw and MHO respondents

Age		YA	MA	EA	ANOVA F value	P value
Oxidative stress markers						
Serum OH Radicals(μmol/L)	MHNO (N=YG+MG+EG =6+35+17)	226±12	255±31	296±32	4.552	0.0148*
	MHOw (N=YG+MG+EG =12+30+18)	240±25	297±54	318±51	13.8	0.0003***
	MHO (N=YG+MG+EG =7+31+20)	401±88	396±41	467±65	3.8	0.0008***
	P value	<0.0001***	<0.0001***	<0.0001***		
Serum FLOP (FIş/ml)	MHNO (N=YG+MG+EG =6+35+17)	147±23	170±17	172±16	4.664	0.0134*
	MHOw (N=YG+MG+EG =12+30+18)	146±14	178±31	188±30	-	0.0007***
	MHO (N=YG+MG+EG =7+31+20)	180±37	190±42	221±46	-	0.018*
	P value	<0.0001***	0.038*	0.041*		
Erythrocytic MDA (nmoles/g Hb)	MHNO	0.65±0.4	0.55±0.1	0.52±0.1	2.44	0.092
	MHOw	0.87±0.7	1.69±0.9	2.36±1	21.68	<0.0001***
	MHO	2.60±0.8	3.29±0.9	3.99±1.1	12.31	<0.0001***
	P value	<0.0001***	<0.0001***	<0.0001***		
Erythrocytic PCO (nmole/g Hb)	MHNO	0.42±0.1	0.47±0.1	0.42±0.1	2.38	0.97
	MHOw	0.43±0.2	0.90±0.5	1.17±0.7	14.96	<0.0001***
	MHO	2.27±1	2.34±0.6	2.88±0.7	6.98	0.0014**

	P value	<0.0001***	<0.0001***	<0.0001***		
Antioxidant Markers						
Erythrocytic CuZn SOD (unit /g Hb)	MHNO	3.30±1	1.48±0.5	2.17±0.7	33.27	<0.0001***
	MHOw	2.84±1.4	2.83±1.5	2.99±1.3	3.49	0.82
	MHO	1.64±0.587	0.53±0.2	0.47±0.1	15.10	<0.0001***
	P value	<0.0001***	<0.0001***	<0.0001***		
Erythrocytic CAT (unit/g Hb)	MHNO	3.01±1.2	3.04±0.9	2.98±0.8	0.033	0.966
	MHOw	3.80±1	2.58±0.9	2.22±0.8	27.03	<0.0001***
	MHO	2.77±0.8	2.42±0.5	1.97±0.6	11.26	<0.0001***
	P value	0.547	<0.0001***	<0.0001***		
Plasma GPX (nmole/min/mg plasma protein)	MHNO	5.76±2.5	5.51±2	4.46±1.4	3.816	0.025*
	MHOw	5.08±0.8	3.63±1.3	2.94±1.2	28.10	<0.0001***
	MHO	5.54±1.7	4.32±1.9	3.82±1.6	4.827	0.010**
	P value	0.792	<0.0001***	<0.0001***		
FRAP (μmole/ml of plasma)	MHNO	4.84±1.2	4.58±1.6	3.86±1.1	3.29	0.041*
	MHOw	5.63±0.9	3.98±1.5	3.19±1.2	28.95	<0.0001***
	MHO	2.96±1.3	3.2±1	2.59±0.7	4.80	0.010*
	P value	<0.0001***	<0.0001***	<0.0001***		
Post hoc Test						
		YA vs MA		YA vs EA		MA vs EA
Serum OH Radicals	MHNO	ns		*		ns
	MHOw	**		***		ns
	MHO	ns		ns		***
Serum FLOP	MHNO	*		*		ns
	MHOw	**		***		ns
	MHO	ns		ns		*
	MHNO	ns		ns		ns

Results and Discussioun

Erythrocytic MDA	MHOw	***	***	***
	MHO	***	***	***
Erythrocytic PCO	MHNO	ns	ns	ns
	MHOw	***	***	***
	MHO	ns	*	**
Erythrocytic CuZn SOD	MHNO	***	***	***
	MHOw	ns	ns	ns
	MHO	***	***	***
Erythrocytic CAT	MHNO	ns	ns	ns
	MHOw	***	***	***
	MHO	***	***	***
Plasma GPX	MHNO	ns	ns	*
	MHOw	***	***	***
	MHO	ns	**	ns
FRAP	MHNO	ns	ns	ns
	MHOw	***	***	***
	MHO	ns	ns	**

All values are presented as mean ±SD. *Data were processed for analysis for one way ANOVA followed by Tukey's test followed by Kruskal Wallis test (Dunns multiple comparisons). One, two and three asterisks signify statistical significance at $p \leq 0.05$, $p \leq 0.005$ and $p \leq 0.0005$ respectively.*

($^\bullet$OH: Hydroxyl Radical, FLOP: Fluorescent Oxidation Products, MDA: Malondialdehyde, PCO: Protein carbonyl, SOD: Superoxide dismutase, FRAP: Ferric reducing ability of plasma, GPX: Glutathione Peroxidase, CAT: Catalase)

It can been seen from Table 4.2.3 that one way ANOVA analysis confirmed that in MHOw and MHO, there was age-wise increase in OS indices, serum OH radicals, FLOP, erythrocytic MDA, PCO, and decrease in antioxidant enzymes, CuZn SOD, CAT, GPx, and total antioxidant capacity indicator, FRAP. However, this pattern is absent or mildly significant in the MHNO group. Further analysis using Tukey's test was performed to assess which pairs of groups are different from each other. The absence of significant changes with age in the MHNO group was clearly indicated, while age related changes were clearly significant between all age groups in the MHOw and MHO groups for all parameters except PCO, GPx and FRAP which did not show significant age related changes in the MHO. This could be attributed to initially high PCO and low FRAP in this group.

This again confirmed that younger MHNO respondents began with a healthy profile which was retained as they aged, while the young MHO began with an unhealthy profile which did not worsen with age. On the other hand, the young MHOw showed a healthy profile which grew towards becoming unhealthy as they aged.

One-way ANOVA was also conducted to assess whether, for each age group, there was a significant difference between MHNO, MHOw and MHO groups. It can be seen that this was indeed the case for all parameters except with regard to initial values of erythrocytic CAT and GPx which did not differ in the Young Adults but differences became statistically significant in the Middle aged Adults and the Elderly.

Table 4.2.4. Age- wise distribution of inflammatory markers in groups of MHNO, MHOw and MHO.

Age		YA	MA	EA	ANOVA	
					F value	P value
Inflammatory markers						
CRP (mg/ml)	MHNO	0.99±0.3	1.12±0.6	0.97±0.6	0.64	0.526
	MHOw	1.11±0.5	1.97± 0.8	2.59±0.8	36.57	<0.0001***
	MHO	2.7±0.9	3.06± 0.7	3.25±0.8	19.6	<0.0001***
	P value	<0.0001***	<0.0001**	<0.0001**		
TNF-α (pg/ml)	MHNO (N=YG+MG+EG=3+22+10)	26.6±16.7	35.8±10.5	31.1±11.9	-	0.308
	MHOw (N=YG+MG+EG=10+14+7)	38±11.5	41.7± 14.9	62.2±19.9	-	0.009**
	MHO (N=YG+MG+EG=4+17+10)	82.3±25.5	93.3± 35.8	131.8±15.5	-	0.007**
	P value	<0.0001	<0.0001*	<0.0001*		

		***	**	**		
IL 6 (pg/ml)	MHNO (N=YG+MG+EG=3+22+10)	5.9±1.7	6.4±1.6	6.2±1.9	-	0.876
	MHOw (N=YG+MG+EG=10+14+7)	7.5±1.2	9.5±1.8	12.8±4.7	-	0.001**
	MHO (N=YG+MG+EG=4+12+8)	16.1±5.2	18.2±3.9	25.1±8.9	-	0.017*
	P value	<0.0001 ***	<0.0001* **	<0.0001* **		

Post hoc Test

		YA vs MA	YA vs EA	MA vs EA
CRP	MHNO	ns	ns	ns
	MHOw	**	***	***
	MHO	***	***	*
TNF –α	MHNO	ns	ns	ns
	MHOw	ns	*	*
	MHO	ns	*	*
IL 6	MHNO	ns	ns	ns
	MHOw	ns	***	*
	MHO	ns	ns	*

All values are presented as mean ±SD. Data were processed for analysis for one way ANOVA followed by Tukey's test followed by Kruskal wallis Test (Dunns multiple comparisons). One, two and three asterisks signify statistical significance at p≤0.05, p≤0.005 and p≤0.0005 respectively.

CRP: C reactive protein, TNF–α: Tumor necrosis factor alpha, IL 6: Interleukin 6.

It can been seen from Table 4.2.4 that one way ANOVA analysis confirmed that in MHOw and MHO, there was age-wise increase in inflammatory markers, CRP, TNF alpha and IL 6. However, this pattern was absent in the MHNO group. Further analysis using Tukey's test was performed to assess which pairs of groups are different from each other. The absence of significant changes with age in the MHNO group was clearly indicated, while CRP showed significant age related changes between all age groups in the MHOw and MHO. TNF alpha and IL 6 showed significant increase from middle age group.

Erythrocytic and plasma oxidative stress markers and antioxidant status for the various age groups of MHNO, MHOw and MHO respondents is presented graphically in Fig 4.2.1, to highlight the different patterns described in the Table 4.2.3 and 4.2.4. It is visible that for all parameters, the healthy profile of the MHNO group shows minimal changes with age. It is also interesting to observe that in the Young Adults, the difference between MHNO and MHOw is minimal, which increases as the age increases, and greater differences are visible in the Middle age and elderly groups. The unhealthy profile of the MHO for all age groups is also clearly visible.

Fig 4.2.1   *(a)*   *(b)*

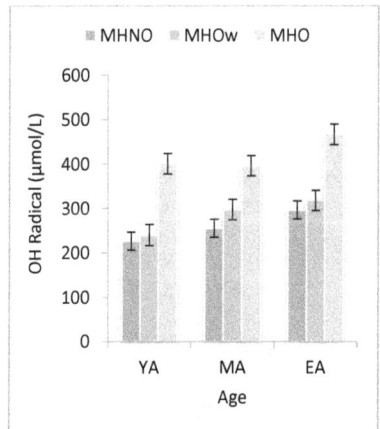
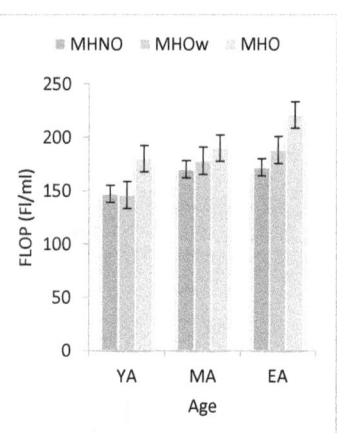

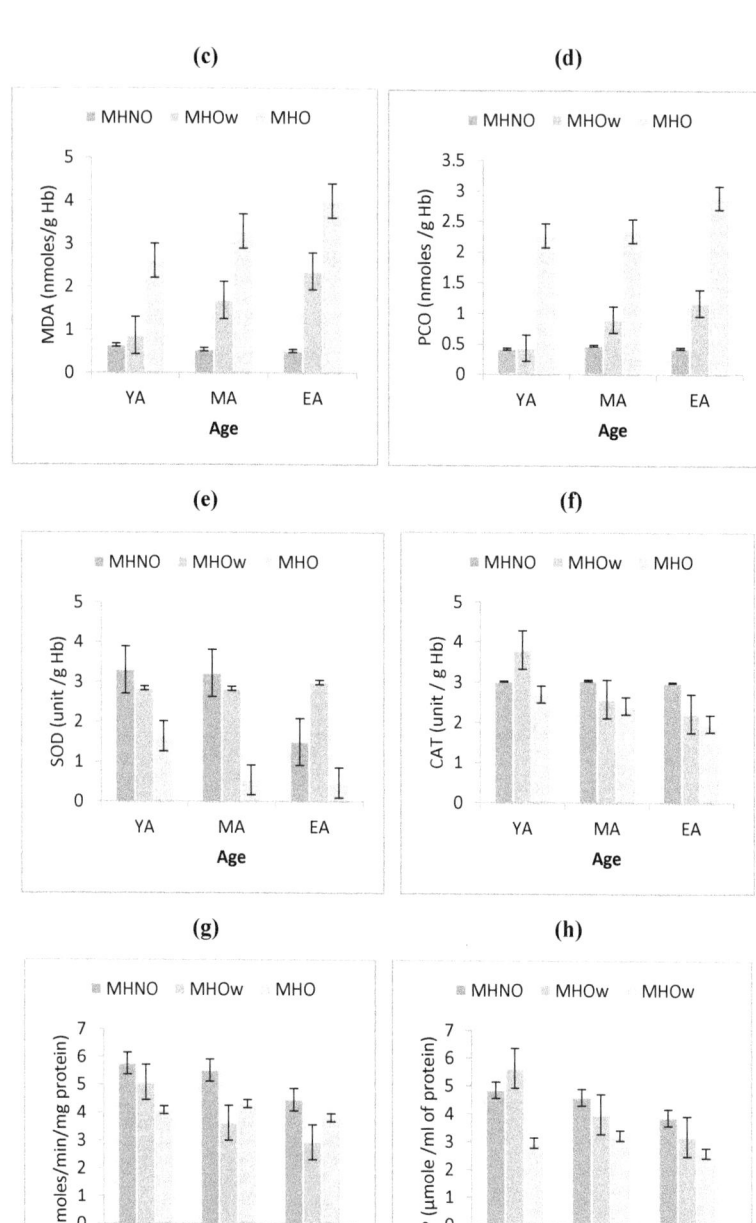

(i)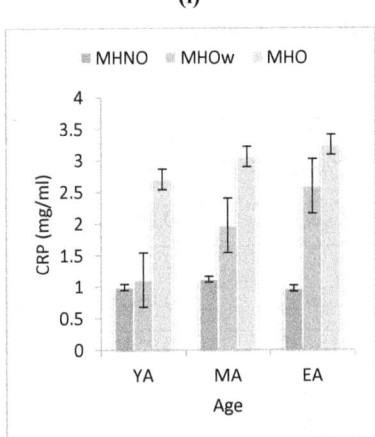

(j)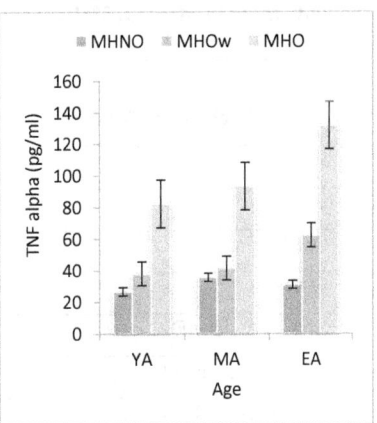

(k)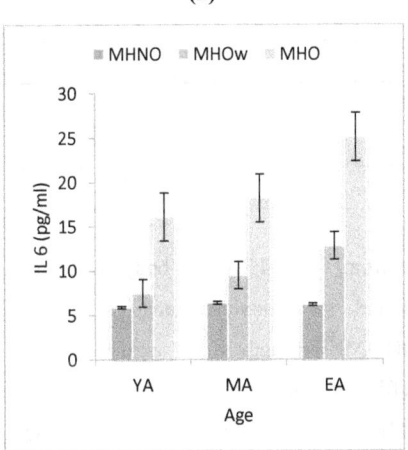

Figure. 4.2.1: Age- wise distribution of (a) OH Radicals, (b) FLOP, (c) MDA, (d) PCO, (e) erythrocytic SOD, (f) erythrocytic CAT, (g) plasma GPx, (h) FRAP, (i) CRP, (j) TNF alpha, (k) IL 6 in MHNO, MHOw and MHO respondents.

The relationship between age and body mass index (BMI), oxidative stress, antioxidant and inflammatory markers, was examined by computing the correlation coefficients and results are presented in Table 4.2.4.

Table 4.2.4. Impact of Age on Body Mass Index, and Oxidative stress (OS) indicators in MHNO, MHOw and MHO respondents.

Biochemical Measures	Age (20-80 year)		
	MHNO	MHOw	MHO
Body Weight	0.266*	0.292*	0.299*
BMI	0.397*	0.533*	0.676*
OH Radical	0.137	0.287*	0.349*
FLOP	0.138	0.280*	0.299*
Erythrocytic MDA	-0.085	0.354*	0.482*
Erythrocytic PCO	-0.135	0.281*	0.351*
Erythrocytic SOD	-0.088	-0.180	-0.223*
Erythrocytic CATALASE	0.063	-0.342*	-0.445*
Plasma GPX	-0.201	-0.217*	-0.252*
FRAP	-0.205*	-0.204 *	-0.211*
CRP	-0.06	0.224*	0.286*
TNF alpha	-0.045	0.238*	0.380*
IL 6	0.035	0.297*	0.616*

It can be seen from Table 4.2.4 that body weight as well as BMI increased with increasing age, and total antioxidant capacity as indexed by FRAP decreased, in all groups, MHNO, MHOw and MHO as indicated by the statistically significant correlation coefficients. However, all other parameters showed significant correlation with age in MHOw and MHO but not in MHNO. Oxidative stress indicators, Erythrocytic MDA and PCO as well as inflammatory markers, CRP, TNF alpha and IL6 correlated positively, and antioxidant enzymes erythrocytic SOD, CAT and plasma GPx, showed negative correlation with age in the MHOw and MHO groups.

The correlations are expressed graphically in Figure 4.2.3 (a) to (k), and confirms visually the pattern described in Table 4.2.3 and 4.2.4.

(a) Age vs OH Radical (b) Age vs FLOP

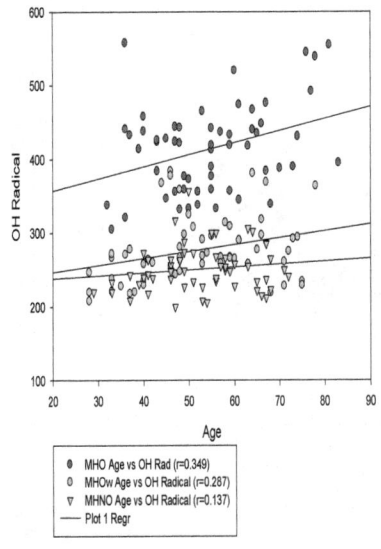

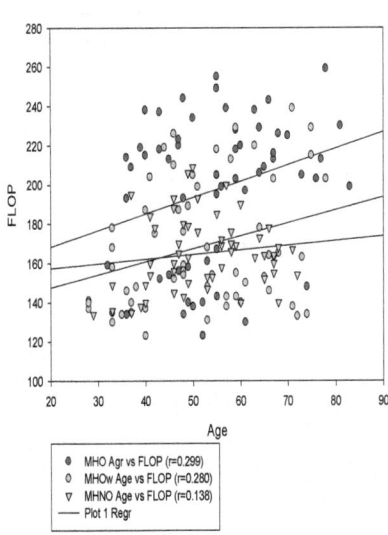

Results and Discussioun

(c) Age vs MDA (d) Age vs PCO

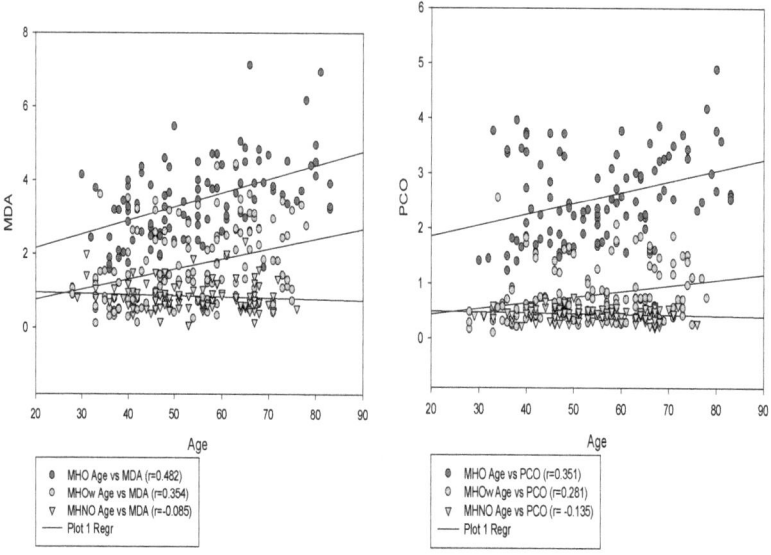

(e) Age vs CuZn SOD (f) Age vs CAT

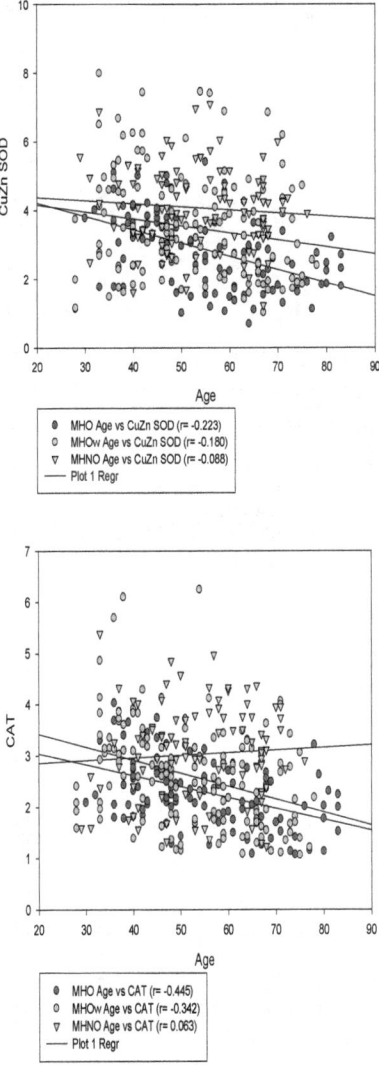

(g) Age vs GPx (h) Age vs FRAP

Results and Discussioun

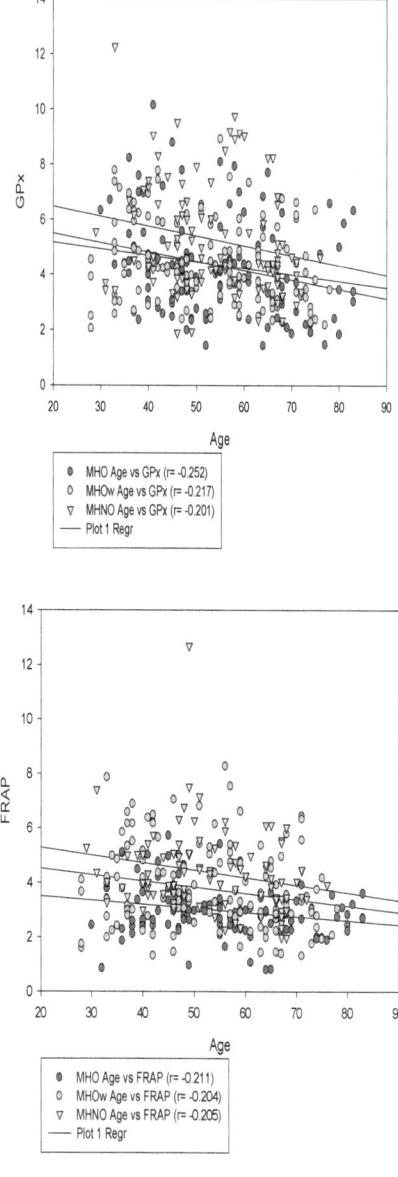

(i) Age vs CRP (j) Age vs TNF alpha

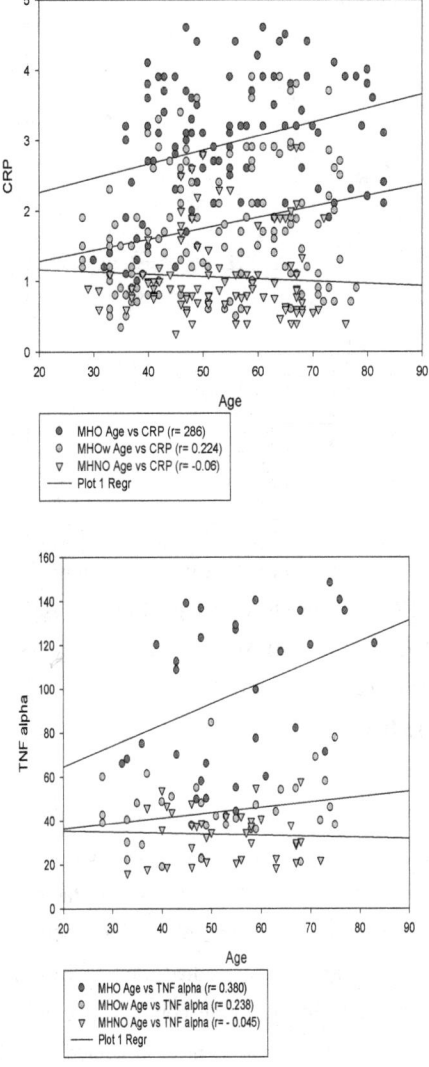

(k) Age vs IL 6

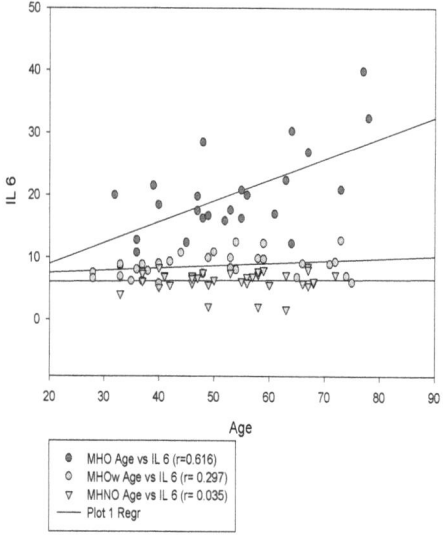

Figure. 4.2.3: depicts the correlation graphs to show differences among MHONO, MHOw and MHO respondents with regard to age vs. OS indices (a) Age vs OH Radicals, (b) Age vs FLOP, (c) Age vs MDA, (d) Age vs PCO, (e) Age vs SOD, (f) Age vs CAT, (g) Age vs GPx, (h) Age vs FRAP, (i) Age vs CRP, (j) Age vs TNF alpha, (k) Age vs IL 6.

Discussion

The present study were designed to investigate the effects of different age groups on various blood parameters like NCEP ATP III risk factors for MetS, oxidative stress and inflammatory markers in MHNO, MHOw and MHO group respondents. In this cross sectional case control study, we had used NCEP ATP III criteria for Met S to define metabolic health in non obese controls, overweight and obese respondents because NCEP ATP III criteria is most accepted in clinical practice to define metabolically healthy obesity (MHO).

The most striking finding of this study is that weight and BMI increases as age advances in all groups of respondents studied. Both age and body weight correlated significantly and consistently with BMI in all study groups, indicating that as age increases the percent body fat increases. This is corroborated by earlier findings observed by our lab. We have reported that in disease free postmenopausal women, age was significantly positively correlated with body weight. [Mittal PC and Kant R., 2009]. Weight gain as a function of age seems to be common among adults [Pi-Sunyer FX et al, 2006], even though it is not acknowledged by Age-Weight normative tables.

All the risk factors of MetS as prescribed by NCEP ATP III namely, waist circumference (WC) fasting plasma glucose (FPG), HDL-C, TG and SBP were found to be in normal range. However, within this normal range, there was statistically significant difference in WC, FBG, TG, HDL-C, SBP, TC, and LDL, but not DBP with age in MHOw but not in MHNO and MHO groups. Tukey's post hoc HSD test revealed that younger aged MHNO respondents began with a healthy profile which was retained as they aged, while the young MHO began with an unhealthy profile which did not worsen with age. The young MHOw respondents showed a healthy metabolic profile which grew towards becoming unhealthy as they aged. It may be inferred from the results that obesity, diabetes and other metabolic disorder is associated with the ageing process [Ahima RS, 2009]. It is well documented in literature that the prevalence rate of obesity and its related metabolic disturbances increases as age advances. [Villareal DT, Apovian CM, Kushner RF et al., 2005]. Many reports confirm that obesity and its related predisposing conditions can accelerate the process of ageing and lead to early mortality [Tzanetakou IP, Katsilambros NL, Benetos A et al, 2012]. None of the studies reported above have been conducted on metabolically healthy respondents. Our study confirms that the pattern reported in MetS is observed even in the metabolically healthy phenotype, even as the parameters remained within the prescribed range.

Recent research has focused on comparing metabolically healthy obesity phenotype with their metabolically unhealthy counterparts. It has been suggested that metabolically healthy obesity (MHO) is a subset of obesity which seems to be protected against obesity related metabolic complications irrespective of higher body weight [Goossens GH., 2017]. Thus a heterogeneous metabolic risk profile might exist among obese respondents. The prevalence rate of obesity phenotypes depends upon race/ethnicity and it has been found variation in MHO phenotypes varies from 1.1 to 28.5% which is largely depend upon diverse definitions to define metabolic health profile used by different research studies or methodological issues [Phillips CM, 2013]. Until now, there are no universally accepted definitions to define MHO phenotype but NCEP ATP III is most acceptable by research community. It has been reported that variation in prevalence rate of MHO and metabolically unhealthy (MUO) phenotype also dependent upon index markers such as BMI and WC. Similar variations are reported in community based population study by Liu et al [Liu C, Wang C, Guan S, et al., 2019] and they found variation from 4.2 to 13.6% in MHO prevalence when it was defined by BMI, while from 14 to 40.2 % when it was defined by WC. Prevalence of metabolically healthy obesity defined by NCEP ATP III is highest in the 45-50 year age groups, and declined thereafter, as determined by BMI but prevalence of WC-defined obesity increased with aging, whilst the age-specific prevalence of BMI defined obesity remained stable before age 65 years and then decreased gradually afterward according to criteria/definitions of both obesity and metabolic abnormalities. MHO might be an intermediate state of MUO, and further study is needed to clarify this issue.

The prevalence of obesity is rapidly increasing worldwide but it is more prevalent in older age groups. Obesity and ageing share similar mechanisms in biochemical predispositions associated with them. An analysis reported that the phase transition from MHO to MUHO phenotype is likely to occur as one moves from younger to older age groups [Arterburn DE, Crane PK, Sullivan SD., 2004]. Hence, it is important in clinical practice to assess biochemical markers in MHO and MUHO phenotype in different age subjects to study differences in the etiology, pathogenesis and related inflammatory pattern and implications.

It is well known that oxidative stress increases as one ages. Hence, we studied the redox homeostasis balance in different age groups of metabolically healthy non obese controls (MHNO), overweight (MHOw) and obese (MHO) respondents of these three age groups. As discussed in Chapter 1, significant difference was observed in MHO group as compared to MHNO with regard to all OS markers while MHOw and

MHNO group did not show significant difference. The oxidative damage indices OH radicals, FLOPs, MDA and PCO were higher in all age groups of MHO as well as MHOw group while the indices of antioxidant enzymes and total antioxidant activity were higher in MHNO group, indicating the MHNO group maintained efficient homeostasis through all ages, but MHOw and MHO showed significant increase in oxidative stress in all age groups.

Increased oxidative stress has been linked to age-related diseases which are associated with obesity [Pi-Sunyer FX., 2006, Ozata M, Mergen M, Oktenli C., et al., 2002], but this does not deal with metabolically healthy obesity. It has been suggested that the MHO subset may be on the way to becoming 'unhealthy' obese due to sudden rise in level of reactive oxygen species that causes ROS induced lipid peroxidation and protein carbonylation [Kramer CK, Zinman B, Retnakaran R., 2013].

It is well accepted that obesity is associated with redox imbalance that appears to induce obesity linked ageing process. It is well known that an increase in reactive oxygen species (ROS) generation during ageing process is a consequence of a decrease in efficacy of antioxidant protection. Our study is primarily focused on impact of ageing on all OS markers in MHNO, MHOw and MHO respondents. It was interesting to find that younger MHNO respondents began with a healthy profile which was retained as they aged, while the young MHO began with an unhealthy profile which did not worsen with age. On the other hand, the young MHOw showed a healthy profile which grew towards becoming unhealthy as they aged. This difference can be explained can be explained by the changes observed in the antioxidant enzymes, SOD and Catalase and GPX and total antioxidant capacity which decreased with age in MHOw while MHO group represent declined level of antioxidants at early stage group.

A similar pattern of worsening with age is evident in the inflammatory markers CRP, TNF alpha and IL 6 in the metabolically healthy overweight and obese groups but no age-related change is evident in the normal weight controls. Obesity is significantly linked to the inflammatory state [Wellen KE and Hotamisligil GS., 2005]. A strong correlation between age and inflammatory markers in MHO represent that as we age there is drastic change in metabolic profile in terms of inflammatory markers that convert the MHO into metabolically unhealthy obesity [Aguilar-Salinas CA, Garcia E, Robles L et al., 2008; Goossens GH, 2017]. Several research studies demonstrated that there is reshuffling of body fat distribution with age which is responsible for generating phenotypic heterogeneity in obesity that leads to development of metabolically healthy and unhealthy phenotypes. [Alam I, Pin Ng T., Larbi A., 2012]. Epidemiological evidence has demonstrated that normal adipose tissue function has been associated to healthier metabolic profile even in obese phenotypes [Bluher M., 2010] while adipose tissue dysfunction especially in case of unhealthy obesity is linked to enhanced expression of TNF alpha, proinflammatory cytokine secretion, activation of macrophages which is associated with obesity comorbidities [Schmidt MI., Duncan BB., Sharrett AR, et al., 1999].

One of the most significant observation from this chapter was that there was no increase in OS with ageing metabolically healthy non obese controls (MHNO), indicating their healthier metabolic profile while there was significant increase in OS and inflammatory markers with age both in MHOw and MHO group. This is contrary to many studies which show an increase in OS and inflammatory markers with age. However, these studies do not assess changes in body weight with age, which also increases as age advances.

Another finding is that the age related pattern observed in MetS is also found in the metabolically healthy phenotype, even as the parameters remained within the prescribed range. All parameters changes only marginally in the overweight group but worsened in the obese.

Chapter 4.3. To assess gender-specific association of NCEP ATP III MetS risk factors, oxidative stress, redox balance and inflammatory markers in metabolically healthy Controls, overweight and obese respondents.

In chapter 4.1, differences with regard to oxidative stress indices and redox balance between metabolically healthy Controls and their overweight counterparts with regard most parameters were minimal, but significant differences were found between overweight and obese groups. Inflammatory markers, CRP, TNF-alpha and IL-6 in all groups were significantly correlated to BMI. The metabolically healthy overweight were more like the Controls while in the obese the pattern was indicative of the breakdown of adaptation leading to more significant redox damage.

These were assessed for age-wise changes in chapter 4.2, and differences were reported describing age-related changes in various phenotypes of metabolically healthy respondents, namely, normal weight, overweight and obese groups with regard to NCEP ATP risk factors for MetS, oxidative stress and redox balance indices and inflammatory markers. It was interesting to observe that all parameters changed only marginally in the overweight group but worsened in the obese.

Gender is a crucial determinant of obesity as well as oxidative stress. The study groups described in Chapter 4.1 were analyzed for gender differences and the findings are presented in this chapter. The general characteristics of a cross section of male and female, presented in Table 4.3.1, confirmed that all the groups were matched for age. The BMI of the males and females of the MHNO groups (Males: 23 ±1.6 and Females: 22.5±1.24), MHOw group (Males: 26.6 ±0.9 and Females: 27.2±1.1) and MHO groups (Males: 32.02±5.4 and Female 33.4±0.9), were also matched.

Table 4.3.1.General characteristics of Male and Female respondents assigned to MHNO, MHOw and MHO.

		MHNO	MHOw	MHO
N	Male	56	74	60
	Female	44	73	42
Age (years)	Male	55.3±11.7	53±14	55.3±13.7
	Female	52.3±10.8	52.6±12.5	55.1±14
Height (cm)	Male	162±7.1	163.8±4.2	165±4.3
	Female	157.4±7.7	153.6±3.3	153±3.3
Weight (Kg)	Male	61.9±6.8	68.9±6.5	86.2±5.4
	Female	56.9±6.7	63.7±5.6	78.1±4.4
BMI (Kg/m^2)	Male	23±1.7	26.6±0.9	32±5.4
	Female	22.5±1.2	27.2±1.1	33.4±0.9

All values are presented as mean ±SD.

All respondents were enrolled after ensuring that they had tested negative for all

NCEP ATP III diagnostic criteria risk factors for metabolic syndrome (Met S) except for body weight and related indices, BMI and waist circumference, and other clinical biochemical measures, to define metabolic health (MH) in MHNO (Male/Female), MHOw (Male/Female) and MHO (Male/Female) respondents [NCEP ATP III, 2010]. However, we have seen in chapters 4.1 and 4.2 that there is gradation in these values within the acceptable range with various BMI groups under investigation. Hence, the data was analyzed in relation to impact of gender, and findings are presented in Table 4.3.2.

Table 4.3.2. Gender wise comparison of risk factors of MetS in metabolically healthy non obese controls (MHNO), MH overweight (MHOw) and MH obese (MHO) respondents.

		MHNO	MHOw	MHO	ANOVA	
					F value	P value
NCEP ATP III Diagnostic Criteria For Met S						
Waist Circumference Men:≥90cm Women :≥80 cm	Male	69.7±4.9	82.8±9.3	91.5±4.8	142.4	<0.0001**
	Female	82.8±6.6	88.6±9.2	113.9±3.7	152.6	<0.0001**
	P value	0.01*	<0.0001**	<0.0001**		
Fasting Plasma Glucose >100 mg/dl	Male	86.2±1.0	92.8±5.8	101.8±9.6	48.6	<0.0001**
	Female	87.7±7.9	93.8±5	103.6±8.8	56.08	<0.0001**
	P value	0.8	0.3	0.34		
Triglycerides ≥150 mg/dl	Male	128±18.7	130.9±6.5	149.6±13.5	45.5	<0.0001**
	Female	131.1±19	132±10.3	156.8±17.6	56.6	<0.0001**
	P value	0.4	0.43	0.003**		
HDL-Cholesterol Men :≤ 40 mg/dl	Male	54.7±6.8	53.3±4.6	50.9±5.9	8.8	0.001**

Women :≤ 50 mg/dl	Female	53.6±7.4	52.9±5.4	46.4±6.5	18.3	<0.0001***
	P value	0.73	0.64	0.004**		
Systolic Blood Pressure Systolic ≥130 mmHg	Male	114±5.2	119±5	124±5	41.5	<0.0001***
	Female	115±5.2	120±3	120±3	20.9	<0.0001***
	P value	0.73	0.60	0.02*		
Other related biochemical measures						
Diastolic Blood Pressure Diastolic ≥80 mmHg	Male	76±6	79±3	81±5	14.8	<0.0001***
	Female	75±7	78±4	79±2	8.8	0.0002***
	P value	0.88	0.42	0.22		
Total Cholesterol 150- 250 mg/dl	Male	175±11.3	180.6±8.9	194.9±12.4	52.4	<0.0001***
	Female	178.7±10	182.6±11.5	207.5±19.4	83.6	<0.0001***
	P value	0.08	0.24	0.008**		
Low Density Lipoprotein ≤150 mg/dl	Male	138±11.4	102.3±10.9	114±13.8	36.4	<0.0001***
	Female	141.5±10	105.7±14	129.7±16.7	59	<0.0001***
	P value	0.07	0.10	<0.0001***		
Tukey's Post hoc Test						
		MHNO vs MHOw	MHNO vs MHO	MHOw vs MHO		
WC	Male	***	***	***		
	Female	***	***	***		
FBG	Male	***	***	***		
	Female	***	***	***		
TG	Male	ns	***	***		

	Female	ns	***	***
HDL	Male	ns	**	*
	Female	ns	***	***
SBP	Male	***	***	**
	Female	***	***	ns
DBP	Male	**	***	ns
	Female	**	***	ns
TC	Male	*	***	***
	Female	ns	***	***
LDL	Male	**	***	***
	Female	*	***	***

All values are presented as mean ±SD. One, two and three asterisks signify statistical significance at p≤0.05, p≤0.005 and p≤0.0005 respectively

Cut-offs prescribed by NCEP-ATP III criteria: Waist circumference (WC): Men :≥90 cm, Women :≥80cm; Plasma fasting glucose (FPG): ≥100 mg/dl; Triglyceride (TG): ≥150 mg/dl, HDL Cholesterol (HDL-C): Men :≤ 40 mg/dl Women :≤ 50 mg/dl; blood pressure (BP): Systolic (SBP) ≥130 mmHg, Diastolic (DBP)>85 mmHg; total cholesterol (TC): 150- 250 mg/dl, low density lipoprotein (LDL-C): ≤150 mg/dl.

It can be seen from Table 4.3.2 that no statistically significant difference is observable in this cross sectional sample in any of lipoprotein fractions, fasting blood glucose, blood pressure except waist circumference in relation to gender in MHNO and MHOw group although females of MHO group appear to have significantly higher triglyceride (TG), total cholesterol (TC), low density lipoproteins (LDL), fasting blood glucose levels and waist circumference than males.

As expected, one way ANOVA confirmed the statistically significant difference in WC, FBG, TG, HDL-C, SBP, DBP, TC, and LDL in male and female in relation to all obesity phenotypes, MHNO, MHOw and MHO groups. No significant gender difference was found in any parameter on comparing pairs of phenotypes on application of Tukey's posthoc test with the possible exception of total cholesterol when MHNO and MHOw are compared and systolic blood pressure on comparing MHOw with MHO. These differences do not conform to any major pattern.

Oxidative stress markers were also compared for gender differences in MHNO, MHOw and MHO respondents and findings are presented in Table 4.3.3.

Table 4.3.3. Gender wise comparisons between males and females of MHNO, MHOw and MHO groups with regard to marker of Erythrocytic and plasma oxidative stress markers, antioxidants and redox status.

Age		MHNO	MHOw	MHO	ANOVA	
					F value	P value
Oxidative stress markers						
Serum OH Radicals(µmol/L)	Male (N=29+30+28)	261±33	276±14	318±51	63.6	<0.0001 ***
	Female (N=27+26+28)	256±32	312±58	407±75	119.8	<0.0001 ***
	P value	0.22	0.010*	<0.0001 ***		
Serum FLOP (FI§/ml)	Male (N=29+30+28)	169±15	163±29	162±30	0.52	0.592
	Female (N=27+26+28)	169±19	188±28	189±44	35.5	<0.0001 ***
	P value	0.89	0.002**	<0.0001 ***		
Erythrocytic MDA (nmoles/g Hb)	Male	0.90±0.4	1.60±0.8	3.18±0.8	155.4	<0.0001 ***
	Female	0.79±0.4	1.88±1.3	3.88±1.3	89.9	<0.0001 ***
	P value	0.16	0.11	0.0008* **		
Erythrocytic PCO (nmole/g Hb)	Male	0.41±0.1	0.84±0.5	2.32±0.7	198.3	<0.0001 ***

	Female	0.48±0.1	0.94±0.7	2.87±0.7	206.5	<0.0001 ***
	P value	0.09	0.37	0.0003**		

Antioxidant Markers

Erythrocytic CuZn SOD (unit /g Hb)	Male	3.87±1.3	3.90±1.7	2.43±1	20.3	<0.0001 ***
	Female	4.29±0.9	4.02±1.7	3.37±0.9	5.2	0.006**
	P value	0.07	0.68	<0.0001**		
Erythrocytic CAT (unit/g Hb)	Male	2.59±0.7	2.46±0.8	2.04±0.6	8.6	0.0003**
	Female	3.57±0.8	2.95±1.2	2.63±0.6	10.5	<0.0001 ***
	P value	0.02*	0.005**	0.01**		
Plasma GPX (nmole/min/mg plasma protein)	Male	4.29±1.5	4.27±1.4	3.62±1.6	3.9	**0.020***
	Female	6.44±2	5.14±1.5	5.26±1.7	8.6	0.0003**
	P value	<0.0001 ***	0.0006**	<0.0001**		
FRAP (µmole/ml of plasma)	Male	4.09±1.7	4.01±1.1	2.57±0.7	28.9	<0.0001 ***
	Female	4.64±0.9	4.10± 1.9	3.52±1	6	0.003**
	P value	0.06	0.74	<0.0001**		

Post hoc Test

		MHNO vs MHOw	MHNO vs MHO	MHOw vs MHO
Serum OH Radicals	Male	ns	***	***
	Female	***	***	***
Serum FLOP	Male	ns	ns	ns
	Female	**	***	***
Erythrocytic MDA	Male	***	***	***
	Female	***	***	***

Erythrocytic PCO	Male	***	***	***
	Female	***	***	***
Erythrocytic CuZn SOD	Male	ns	***	***
	Female	ns	**	*
Erythrocytic CAT	Male	ns	***	***
	Female	**	***	ns
Plasma GPX	Male	ns	*	*
	Female	***	**	ns
FRAP	Male	ns	***	***
	Female	ns	**	ns

All values are presented as mean ±SD. Data were processed for analysis for pared t test followed by Mann Whitney Test for non parametric data sets. One, two and three asterisks signify statistical significance at $p \leq 0.05$, $p \leq 0.005$ and $p \leq 0.0005$ respectively.

(•OH: Hydroxyl Radical, FLOP: Fluorescent Oxidation Products, MDA: Malondialdehyde, PCO: Protein carbonyl, SOD: Superoxide dismutase, FRAP: Ferric reducing ability of plasma, GPX: Glutathione Peroxidase, CAT: Catalase)

The data were assessed to investigate the gender wise differences with regard to OS markers with regard to phenotype. No significant gender differences were seen in MHNO group with regard to any OS indices except GPx, and in MHOw group, no gender difference was visible with regard to erythrocytic parameters MDA, PCO and CuZn SOD, as well total antioxidant capacity as indexed by FRAP, while all OS indices show a gender difference in the MHO group. Interestingly, in this group, females have a higher level of OS indices OH radicals, FLOP, MDA and PCO, but they also have a higher level of antioxidant enzymes, CuZn SOD, CAT, GPx and consequently a higher total antioxidant capacity measured by FRAP. The overall pattern is indicative of better adaptation and restoration of homeostasis in the obese females as compared to the male counterparts.

Since BMI is used to grade the respondents into the three phenotypes under study, applying one-way ANOVA to phenotype confirmed its significant impact in males as well as females on all indicators of OS, namely serum hydroxyl radicals, FLOP, and erythrocytic MDA, PCO, which increased as BMI increased, as well as on antioxidant enzymes, Cu-Zn SOD, CAT, and plasma GPx, and consequently on FRAP.

Further analysis to assess pairwise comparisons between phenotypes, conducted by applying Tukey's post hoc test indicated that except for serum FLOP in males and CAT, GPx and FRAP in females, all indices were statistically significantly different in MHOw and MHO. Differences between MHNO and MHO were significant between males and females with regard to MDA, PCO, but not SOD and FRAP. Gender difference is seen between OH radical, FLOP, CAT, GPx which are significantly different in females but not males. The differences between MHNO and MHO are significant for all parameters for males as well as females. Since FRAP does not differ significantly in males and females when MHNO and MHOw are compared it is indicated that there may be differences in the mechanism of adaptation in males and females but these two phenotypes, namely MHNO and MHOw are more similar to each other than MHOw and MHO.

Table 4.3.4: Gender wise comparisons between male and female of MHNO, MHOw and MHO group with regard to inflammatory markers

Age		MHNO	MHOw	MHO	ANOVA	
					F value	P value
Inflammatory markers						
CRP (mg/ml)	Male	1.1±0.6	2.0±0.8	3.12±0.9	89.9	<0.0001***
	Female	0.9±0.4	1.9± 1.1	3.05±0.6	67.4	<0.0001***
	P value	0.07	0.80	0.71		
TNF –α (pg/ml)	Male (N=15+19+12)	33.1±10.2	42.5±15.5	70.1±11.9	-	<0.0001***
	Female (N=21+9+12)	36.5±8.9	44.2± 16.5	90.6±16.4	-	<0.0001***
	P value	0.19	0.78	<0.0001***		
IL 6 (pg/ml)	Male (N=15+19+12)	6.2±1.9	8.3±1.8	13.4±3.9	-	<0.0001***

	Female (N=21+9+12)	6.4±1.4	9.9± 1.7	16.8±4.0	-	<0.0001***
	P value	0.65	0.05	0.048*		

Post hoc Test

		MHNO vs MHOw	MHNO vs MHO	MHOw vs MHO
CRP	Male	***	***	ns
	Female	***	***	***
TNF –α	Male	ns	***	***
	Female	ns	***	**
IL 6	Male	ns	ns	**

All values are presented as mean ±SD. Data were processed for analysis for one way ANOVA followed by Tukey's test followed by Kruskalwallis Test (Dunns multiple comparisons). One, two and three asterisks signify statistical significance at $p \leq 0.05$, $p \leq 0.005$ and $p \leq 0.0005$ respectively.

(CRP: C reactive protein, TNF–α: Tumor necrosis factor alpha, IL 6: Interleukin 6)

It can be seen from Table 4.3.4 that there is no difference between male and female levels of inflammatory markers CRP, TNF alpha and IL6 in any of the phenotypes, except with regard to TNF –α in MHO, where females had significantly higher levels. A similar gender difference, though less prominent was visible in IL6 levels also. One way ANOVA analysis revealed that male and female of all three groups showed significant increase in inflammatory markers, CRP, TNF alpha and IL 6 as BMI increases across phenotypes.

To assess the relative impacts of body weight and BMI on OS and inflammatory markers, the correlation between BMI and OS markers were calculated and are presented in Table 3.4.

Table 4.3.4. Interrelationships between oxidative stress (OS) markers, body weight and body mass index (BMI), in male and female respondents of MHNO, MHOw and MHO.

		OH Rad	FLOP	MDA	PCO	CuZn SOD	CAT	GPx	FRAP	CRP	TNF alpha	IL6
B M I	MHNO M	0.189	0.174	-0.28	-0.08	-0.041	-0.148	0.082	-0.145	0.066	0.204	0.199
	MHNO F	0.181	0.211	0.075	-0.04	0.07	-0.02	-0.028	0.06	-0.004	0.016	0.192
	MHOw M	0.510	0.557	0.245	0.235	-0.299	-0.143	-0.163	-0.266	0.228	0.248	0.604
	MHOw F	0.360	0.331	0.145	0.141	-0.192	-0.05	-0.12	-0.12	0.213	0.274	0.308
	MHO M	0.204	0.395	0.478	0.287	-0.616	-0.504	0.017	-0.388	-0.013	0.358	0.218
	MHO F	0.666	0.497	0.713	0.609	-0.669	-0.539	0.674	-0.665	0.186	0.484	0.503

Values marked with asterisk are statistically significant at $p \leq 0.05$

It can be seen from Table 4.3.4 that the BMI of MHNO males and females did not show significant correlation with any of OS markers. In the MHOw males, all four OS indices, OH radicals, FLOP, MDA and PCO increased, accompanied with significant decline in CuZn

SOD and consequently a low FRAP as BMI increased, but this pattern was not found in MHOw females, except in the serum parameters OH and FLOP. This indicated that females of MHOw phenotype were not affected to any significant extent with BMI. However, in the MHO the overall pattern was similar in the males and females, showing a significant dependence on BMI with significant increase in all OS indices and decline in antioxidant enzymes and consequent decline in FRAP with BMI.

No significant gender difference was observed in the correlations between BMI and the three inflammatory markers, CRP, TNF alpha and IL6 in any of the metabolically healthy phenotypes. As described in Chapter 4.1, the impact of BMI in the obese group was maximum on TNF alpha and IL6.

Discussion

The present chapter investigated sex wise differences with regard to oxidative stress markers, antioxidant enzymes and inflammation for early diagnosis of obesity to reduce the risk of associated metabolic complications. Gender is an important determinant of many diseases in terms of prevalence, complexity, severity and outcome. The study groups described in Chapter 4.1 were analyzed for gender differences in various phenotypes of metabolically healthy respondents, namely, normal weight, overweight and obese groups with regard to NCEP ATP III risk factors for MetS, oxidative stress and redox balance indices and inflammatory markers and the findings are presented in this chapter. Weight gain as a function of age seems to be common among adults, and has been found to be more for women than for men [Pi-Sunyer FX., 1999]. Weight gain with menopause has been reported in several studies [Wing RR, Matthews KA, Kuller LH, et al., 1991; Pasquali R, Casimirri LF, Labate AMM, et al. 1995], the reason for which may be falling levels of estrogen [Yagi K., 1997; Ruiz-Larrea MB, Martin C, Martinez R, et al., 2000] which causes lowering of basal metabolic rate.

In general, obesity is one of the most important risk factor of metabolic syndrome, cardiovascular diseases and increased mortality. However, impact of obesity may differ from disease risk due to gender, age and metabolic health status. A different phenotype of obese individuals known as metabolically healthy obesity (MHO) seems to represent healthier metabolic profile [Goossens GH., 2017] because MHO individuals are at increased (cardio) metabolic disease risk and type 2 diabetes and may have other comorbidities. [Gaita D, Mosteoru S., 2017]. Therefore, it has been suggested that metabolic phenotyping of obese persons gives perceptive of pathophysiology associated with obesity to identify the high risk subgroups that may help in optimization of prevention and management strategies to combat type 2 diabetes mellitus.

Epidemiologic studies suggest that prevalence rate of overweight and obesity among men and women varies by region. In general, women tend to have higher prevalence rate for obesity (16 %) than men (12 %), whereas the prevalence of overweight is greater for males (24 %) than females (21 %) [Ogden CL, Carroll MD, Curtin LR, et al., 2006]. The gender wise disparities in prevalence rate is primarily associated with pattern of body fat distribution and adipose tissue storage. It is well known that sex hormones play a pivotal role in adipose tissue deposition, distribution, energy balance and metabolism especially female hormone estrogen which have both antioxidant and anti-inflammatory properties. [Giordano S, Hage FG, Xing D, et al., 2015]. It has been reported that menopause affects body fat distribution that may increase the risk of weight gain (obesity) on health. It has also been reported that SOD, CAT decreased and MDA increased with increase in both age and body weight. The changes were more pronounced between premenstrual and postmenstrual groups than normally menstruating control and premenstrual group [Mittal PC, and Kant R., 2009]. It has been also reported that menopause affects body fat distribution that may increase the risk of weight gain (obesity) on health. Beigh et al (2012) [Beigh SH and Jain S., 2012] reported that females have higher incidence of metabolic syndrome (MetS) due to more central obesity. Central obesity has been reported as important risk factor in the development of the MetS and appears to precede the appearance of the other MetS components [Cameron AJ, Boyko EJ, Sicree RA, et al., 2008]. Consistent with previous reports [Cameron AJ, Boyko EJ, Sicree RA et al., 2008], we observed significantly higher waist circumference of the females of metabolically healthy non obese controls (MHNO), overweight (MHOw) and obese (MHO) as compared to their male counterparts, indicating the predisposition of metabolically healthy females to central obesity associated comorbidities. Moreover, the males and females of our three study groups were matched for BMI. We did not find any significant difference between males and females of MHNO and MHOw group with regard to markers of fasting blood glucose, triglyceride, total cholesterol, HDL, LDL and SBP. However, genderwise significant difference was observed in MHO group. Our findings are corroborated by Kim et al [Kim IY, Han KD, Kim DH., et al., 2019] who observed that women with general obesity or MetS showed increased risk of hyperurecemia four times more than males.

As described in previous chapters, we have assessed the systemic redox status in the three study groups of both genders. Some interesting gender differences have emerged from our study. No significant pattern was observed in gender differences with regard to oxidative stress markers OH radicals, FLOP, MDA PCO, antioxidant enzymes CuZn SOD, CAT, GPx, FRAP and consequent redox balance between the metabolically healthy normal weight (MHNO) and overweight (MHOw) respondents. In their obese (MHO) counterparts, however, all OS indices were higher in females, but they also had a higher level of antioxidant enzymes, and consequently a higher total antioxidant capacity. This was an important finding because it indicated better adaptation and restoration of homeostasis in the overweight obese females. However, conflicting results are reported in genderwise studies with regard to oxidative stress markers. Brunelli et al reported [Brunelli E, Domanico F, La Russa D, et al., 2014] significant difference in oxidative stress between the sexes whereas, no difference was found in the total antioxidant capacity. The study further reported that sexwise differences can be explained on the basis of hormonal status especially estrogen level. Despite having strong antioxidant estrogen, females have higher oxidative stress than counterpart males reported by this study. Our findings are further corroborated by Kowalska et al [Kowalska K. and Milnerowicz H. 2016] who found no significant gender difference in MDA, GGT activity (Gamma-glutamyl transpeptidase), and Cu concentrations in healthy subjects aged 20 to 25 years and also reported significantly higher oxidative stress markers in healthy women than men belonging to middle age groups. One recent study showed [Tian S., Liu Y., Feng Ao., et al., 2020] that the females of MHO phenotype group was positively correlated with the risk of hyperurecemia after adjusting confounding variables while this correlation was lacking in MHO males, indicating the favorable metabolic profile of MHO males. Some animal studies reported that the level of oxidative stress was higher in male rats than female rats [Barp J, Araujo AS, Fernandes TR, et al., 2002].

Thus, gender difference is present in many metabolic diseases but their nature and impact on redox homeostasis status needed further evaluation especially in case of metabolically healthy obesity (MHO). None of the parameters showed any significant gender difference with increasing BMI in the normal weight phenotype, while males but not females of the overweight metabolically healthy phenotype were affected, but, in the MHO phenotype, the overall pattern was similar in the males and females, showing a significant dependence on BMI with significant increase in all OS indices and decline in antioxidant enzymes and consequent decline in FRAP with BMI. Previous independent studies demonstrated higher levels of oxidative stress markers in females as compared to males [Fukui T, Yamauchi K, Maruyama M., et al., 2011]. The high BMI and WC in females enrolled in our study may explain this increase in oxidative stress response as compared to males. Yet, it is generally accepted that the prevalence of CVD is higher in males and postmenopausal females [Marie C., 2005] due to hormonal differences and protection provided to premenopausal women by estrogen.

Similarly, no major gender difference was apparent with regard to the inflammatory markers studied in the MHNO and MHOw phenotypes, but in the MHO groups, females had higher TNF $-\alpha$ and, to some extent IL6 also. Our results are confirmed by earlier clinical studies which are related to gender differences in terms of inflammatory markers and immune response against different stressors [Casimir GJA and Duchateau J., 2011; Valentine RJ, McAuley E, Vieira VJ, et al., 2009]. Previous studies reported that women have higher level of inflammatory markers like CRP which is advantageous to women's health during immune response but could be detrimental in case of chronic inflammation [Valentine RJ, McAuley E, Vieira VJ, et al., 2009]. Several studies reported women exhibit greater changes in functioning of immune response against psychological stressors than men [Casimir GJA and Duchateau J., 2011]. The gender difference in immune functioning may be attributed to a variety of factorsin which sex hormones especially estrogen is very important [Cushman M. 2002]. A study conducted on healthy prepubescent children reported that female children suffering from prolonged fever periods have higher level of three cytokines (IL 1, IL 6 and TNF alpha) [Casimir GJA, Heldenbergh F., Hanssens L., et al., 2010]. The main conclusion that emerges from this study is that gender differences in redox mechanisms are apparent in the metabolically healthy overweight groups which is responsible for better homeostasis in the females than males, but the gender difference disappears in the obese groups. Obesity affects both these groups adversely.

Chapter 4.4: To compare metabolically healthy (MH) non obese Controls (MHNO), and those with General Obesity (MHGO) or Central Obesity (MHCO) with regard to NCEP ATP III MetS risk factors, markers of oxidative stress, redox balance and inflammation.

In the foregoing chapters, we have described the biochemical issues related to NCEP ATP III risk factors for MetS, oxidative stress indices and redox balance, and inflammatory markers of metabolically healthy normal weight, overweight and obese respondents who are categorized on the basis of their body mass index. However, all individuals with similar BMI do not have the same distribution of body fat. The main categories of body fat distribution are accumulated fat around the waist, designated Central Obesity and a more generalized fat distribution categorized as General Obesity. In this section, the metabolically healthy (MH) respondents have been categorized into three groups; non obese Controls (MHNO), and those with General Obesity (MHGO) or those with Central Obesity (MHCO), and they are compared with regard to NCEP ATP III risk factors, markers of oxidative stress, redox balance and inflammation.

The general characteristics of the respondents are described in Table 4.4.1. The MHGO and MHCO groups had similar BMI, while the MHNO group was selected with BMI in normal range of 18-25. All the groups were matched for age, height and gender distribution. The MHGO and MHCO groups did not differ with regard to body weight and BMI.

Table 4.4.1: General characteristics of MHNO and respondents suffering from metabolically healthy General Obesity (MHGO) and Central Obesity (MHCO) groups.

Demographic Data	MHNO	MHGO	MHCO
N	100	71	77
Age (years)	53.9±10.23	53.55±11.1	56.12±11.2
Height (cm)	160.1±7.69	160±6.1	157.7±6.4
Weight (kilogram)	59.7±7.23	67.9±9.2	68.77±7.8
Body Mass Index (Kg/m^2)	22.8±0.1	26.4±0.6	27.51±0.9

All values are expressed as Mean ± SD.

Revised NCEP ATP III diagnostic criteria for metabolic syndrome (Met S) and other clinical biochemical measures, to define metabolic health (MH) in MHNO, MHGO and MHCO groups and results are presented in Table 4.4.2.

Table 4.4.2: NCEP ATP III prescribed diagnostic measures and other clinical biochemical measures of MHNO, General obesity (MHGO) and Central obesity (MHCO) groups.

	MHNO	MHGO	MHCO	F value	P value
NCEP ATP III Diagnostic Criteria For Met S					
Waist circumference	75.4±8.02	77.1±2.4	94.2±3.8	241.6	<0.0001***
Fasting Plasma Glucose	86.9±9.1	93.2±5	94.5±7.5	28.2	<0.0001***
Triglyceride	130±18.8	127.8±6.2	136±7.5	7.1	0.006**
HDL-Cholesterol	54.2±7.1	53.4±3.2	48.6±3.9	25	<0.0001***
Systolic Blood Pressure	115±5.22	119.9±5.1	120.3±4.5	29.5	<0.0001***
Diastolic Blood Pressure	75±7.2	79.4±3.3	78.8±4.9	8.4	<0.0001***
Other related biochemical measures:					
Total Cholesterol	176±10.7	178.4±8.6	186.9±9	25.2	<0.0001***
Low density lipoprotein-C	83.8±19.3	142±8.2	149.9±8.7	239.7	<0.0001***
Post hoc Analysis by Tukey's HSD Test					
	MHNO vs MHGO	MHNO vs MHCO	MHGO vs MHCO		
WC	ns	***	***		
FPG	***	***	***		
TG	ns	**	**		
HDL-C	ns	***	***		
SBP	***	***	ns		
DBP	**	**	ns		
TC	ns	***	***		
LDL-C	***	***	*		

All the values are expressed as mean±SD. $p<0.05$, ** $p<0.001$, *** $p<0.0001$. ns: not significant.

(Cut-offs prescribed by NCEP-ATP III criteria: Waist circumference (WC): Men :≥90 cm, Women :≥80cm; Plasma fasting glucose (FPG): ≥100 mg/dl; Triglyceride (TG): ≥150 mg/dl, HDL Cholesterol (HDL-C): Men :≤ 40 mg/dl Women :≤ 50 mg/dl; blood pressure (BP): Systolic (SBP) ≥130 mmHg, Diastolic (DBP) >85 mmHg; total cholesterol (TC): 150- 250 mg/dl, low density lipoprotein (LDL-C): ≤150 mg/dl.)

As dictated by the inclusion criteria, it was ensured that all the metabolic syndrome diagnostic measures and other related biochemical measures do not fall outside the reference range as stated in the NCEP-ATP III norms, except for waist circumference. According to this criterion overweight/obese respondents are metabolically healthy with one risk factor while MHNO Controls are metabolically normal without any risk factor. However, One-way ANOVA confirmed that there was statistically significant difference among the groups at $p < 0.05$ for all risk factors, with the MHCO showing more aberration than the MHGO, while, as expected the MHNO had the healthier metabolic profile.

Since one way ANOVA does not tell which pairs of groups are different from each other, Tukey's post hoc HSD test was performed. It was found that MHGO did not differ significantly from MHNO with regard to waist circumference, despite a higher BMI. MHGO also did not have significant different levels of triglycerides, HDL-C and total cholesterol, but their fasting plasma glucose, systolic and diastolic blood pressure and LDL-C were significantly higher. On the other hand, MHCO differed from MHNO with regard to all risk factors and other related biochemical measures. MHGO and MHCO differed from each other with regard to all parameters except blood pressure.

Plasma/serum OS markers: serum hydroxyl radical ($^{\bullet}OH$), plasma fluorescent oxidation products (FLOP), GPx, FRAP, erythrocytic oxidative stress markers: MDA, PCO, SOD, catalase and circulating (serum) inflammatory markers: C-reactive protein (CRP), tumor necrosis factor alpha (TNF $-\alpha$), interleukin 6 (IL- 6) were assessed in the three groups and results are presented in Table 4.4.3.

Table 4.4.3: Plasma and Erythrocytic oxidative stress markers, and circulating inflammatory markers in respondents of metabolically healthy non obese (MHNO), MHGO and MHCO groups.

Biochemical Markers	MHNO	MHGO	MHCO	ANOVA F Value	p Value
Plasma Oxidative stress markers					
˙OH Radicals (μmol/L) (n=30+29+29)	256±32	265±30	346±42	56.8	<0.0001***
Plasma FLOP (FIş/ml) (n=30+29+29)	169±19	175±29	198±26	23.3	<0.0001***
FRAP (μmole/ml of plasma)	4.33±1.4	3.92±1.2	3.08±1.2	19.5	<0.0001***
Plasma GPX (nmole/min/mg plasma protein)	5.25±2	4.32±1.2	3.15±1.4	36.7	<0.0001***
Erythrocytic Antioxidant Markers					
MDA (nmoles/g Hb)	0.85±0.4	1.67±0.7	2.26±0.9	96	<0.0001***
PCO (nmoles/g Hb)	0.44±0.1	0.65±0.6	1.17±0.7	67.5	<0.0001***
CuZn SOD (unit /g Hb)	4.06±1.2	3.89±0.8	2.88±1.1	29.1	<0.0001***
CAT (unit/g Hb)	3.03±0.9	2.89±0.8	2.22±0.8	20.9	<0.0001***
Serum Inflammatory Markers					
CRP (mg/ml)	1±0.5	1.4±0.6	2.5±0.8	97.5	<0.0001***
TNF –α (pg/ml) (n=22+17+14)	35.4±10	66.8±9.4	119±17.6	168.4	<0.0001***

IL 6 (pg/ml) (n=22+17+14)	6.3±1.6	7.9±1.6	10.6±1.3	38.1	<0.0001***

Post hoc Analysis by Tukeys HSD Test			
	MHNO vs MHGO	**MHNO vs MHCO**	**MHGO vs MHCO**
˙OH Radicals	ns	***	***
FLOP	ns	***	*
FRAP	*	***	***
GPx	***	***	*
MDA	ns	***	***
PCO	*	***	***
CuZn SOD	*	***	***
CAT	ns	***	***
CRP	***	***	***
TNF α	***	***	***
IL 6	***	***	***

All the values are expressed as mean±SD. $p<0.05$, ** $p<0.001$, *** $p<0.0001$. ns: not significant.*

(˙OH: Hydroxyl Radical, FLOP: Fluorescent Oxidation Products, MDA: Malondialdehyde, PCO: Protein carbonyl, SOD: Superoxide dismutase, FRAP: Ferric reducing ability of plasma, GPX: Glutathione Peroxidase, CAT: Catalase, CRP: C reactive protein, TNF–α: Tumor necrosis factor alpha, IL 6: Interleukin 6.)

One-way ANOVA showed highly significant difference ($p<0.0001$) with regard to all oxidative stress markers, antioxidant enzymes, total antioxidant activity, as well as inflammatory marker under study. However, a closer look to the data indicated that the difference between groups were not all significantly different from each other. To serve this purpose we performed Tukey's HSD post hoc analysis to determine pairwise statistical differences. A mild difference at $p<0.05$ was obtained with regard to FRAP, PCO and CuZn SOD between MHNO and MHGO respondents whereas no significant difference was obtained with regard to ˙OH, FLOP, MDA and CAT. On the other hand, there was significant difference between MHNO and MHCO, and between MHCO and MHGO with regard to all parameters under study.

Oxidative damage to erythrocytic membrane by lipid peroxidation and protein carbonylation was evident in both MHGO and MHCO groups, as indicated by the significantly higher (p<0.0001) levels of MDA and PCO as compared to Controls while plasma oxidative stress markers in terms of hydroxyl ($^{\cdot}$OH) radicals, FLOP were significantly (p<0.0001) different in both MHGO and MHCO from MHNO.

Inflammatory markers CRP, TNF alpha, and IL- 6 were significantly (p<0.0001) different from each other, as indicated by one-way ANOVA as well as by Tukey's test for pairwise analysis between groups.

The quantum of difference was more between MHCO and MHNO, and between MHCO and MHGO than that between MHGO and MHNO for all parameters as is evident from figure 4.4.1 (a), (b) and (c), which represent the relative per cent difference of biochemical parameters between different pairs of groups, indicating a greater impact of central obesity than of general obesity on all parameters under study. It was interesting to observe that respondents of the MHGO group were more similar to the MHNO than to the MHCO group.

Fig 4.4.1:   (a)   (b)

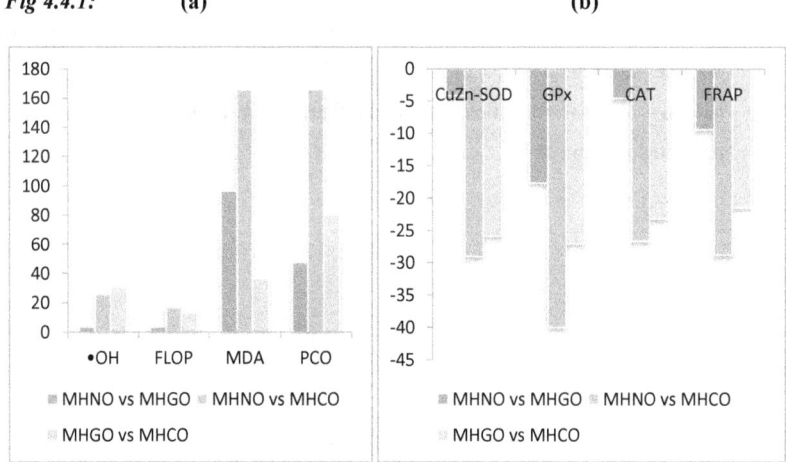

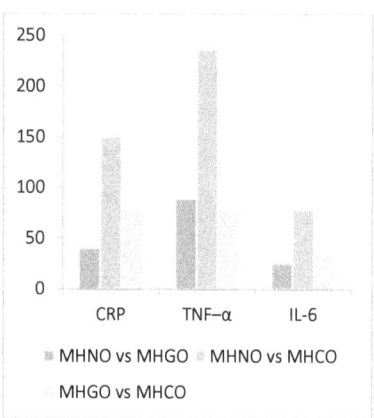

Figure 4.4.1: Relative per cent difference of biochemical parameters between MHNO and MHGO, MHNO and MHCO, and MHCO and MHGO, with regard to (a) serum hydroxyl radicals ('OH), plasma fluorescent oxidation products (FLOP), malondialdehyde (MDA) and protein carbonyl (PCO), (b) CuZn Superoxide dismutase (CuZn SOD), glutathione peroxidase (GPx), catalase (CAT) and ferric reducing ability of plasma (FRAP), and (c) C reactive protein (CRP), tumor necrosis factor alpha (TNF –α), interleukin 6 (IL- 6).

Since the classification of obese into MHGO and MHCO was on the basis of BMI and WC, the interrelationships, as indicated by Pearson's correlation coefficients r, among oxidative stress (OS), antioxidants and inflammatory markers were calculated and are presented in Table 4.4.

Table 4.4.4: Interrelationships among oxidative stress (OS), antioxidants and inflammatory markers with body mass index (BMI) and waist circumference (WC), as indicated by Pearson's correlation coefficientsr.

		˙OH Rad	FLOP	MDA	PCO	SOD	CAT	GPx	FRAP	CRP	TNF	IL 6
BMI	MHNO	0.048	0.016	-0.130	-0.115	-0.234*	-0.118	-0.065	-0.134	0.07	-0.166	0.013
	MHGO	0.266*	0.218	0.238*	.281*	-0.174	-0.195	-0.118	-0.228*	0.228*	0.366*	0.291*
	MHCO	0.192	0.206	0.234*	0.248*	-0.112	-0.107	-0.122	-0.212	0.169	0.207	0.181
WC	MHNO	0.088	0.064	0.038	0.195	0.035	-0.124	-0.083	0.029	-0.165	0.177	0.159
	MHGO	0.244*	0.289*	0.228*	0.295*	-0.223	-0.279*	-0.271*	-0.115	0.169	0.307*	0.281*
	MHCO	0.517*	0.492*	0.643*	0.395*	-0.226*	-0.349*	-0.344*	-0.508*	0.460*	0.488*	0.417*

* indicates statistical significance at p<0.05.

As seen from Table 4.4.4, none of the parameters showed any significant relationship with BMI or WC in the healthy non-obese Controls, except some decline in SOD with increasing BMI.

In MHCO group, all OS and inflammatory markers correlated significantly with waist circumference while only PCO and MDA increased with BMI, but in the MHGO group, the correlations of most parameters significantly correlated with BMI as well as waist circumference.

In both MHGO and MHCO groups, ˙OH radical, FLOP, MDA, PCO and inflammatory markers CRP, TNF alpha, IL-6 increased significantly with increasing BMI. On the other hand, antioxidant enzymes SOD, GPx, CAT and FRAP showed weak correlation with BMI in both groups. However, the relationship was more marked with WC. As WC increased, OS markers ˙OH radical, FLOP, MDA, PCO and inflammatory markers CRP, TNF alpha, IL 6 showed significant positive relationship, and negative relationship with antioxidant enzymes in both groups. The relationship among increasing OS, inflammation and decreasing antioxidant capacity is more in central obesity group which indicated that the effect of WC on prooxidant-antioxidant balance as well as on inflammation is more pronounced than that of BMI.

Fig 4.4.2 (a) OH Rad vs WC (b). FLOP vs WC

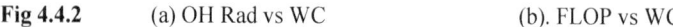

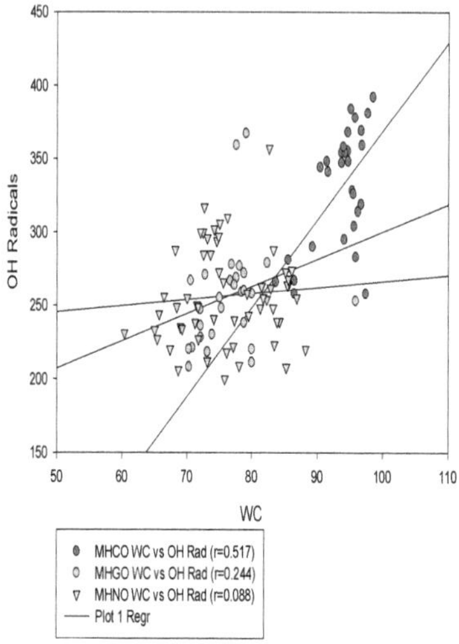

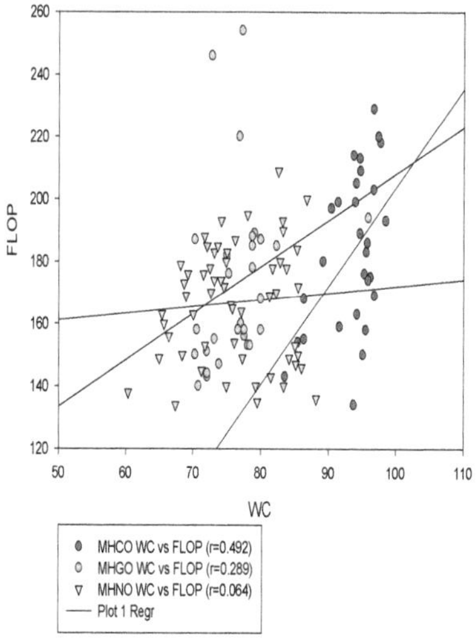

(c) MDA vs WC (d). PCO vs WC

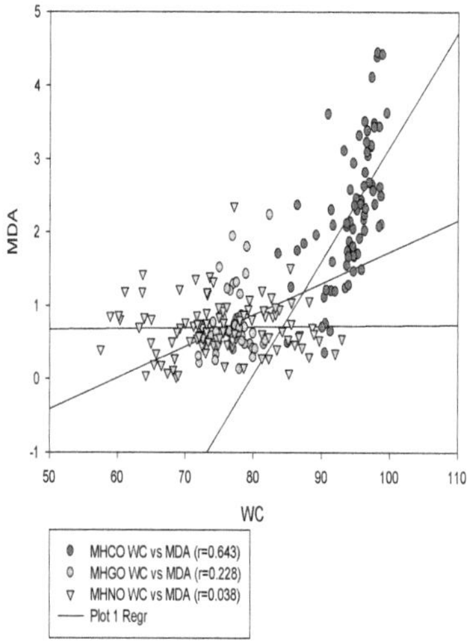

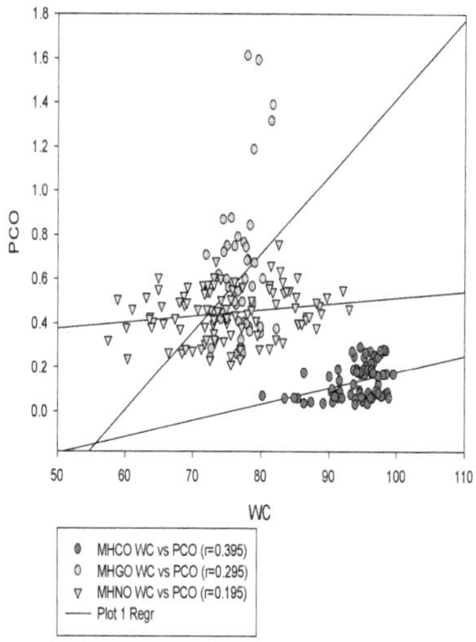

(e). CuZn SOD vs WC (f). CAT vs WC

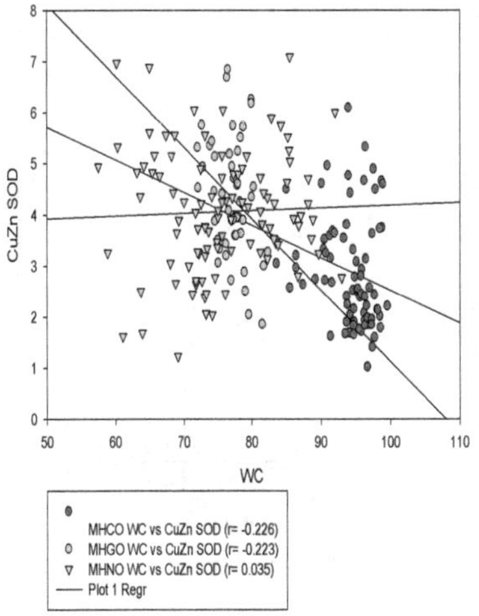

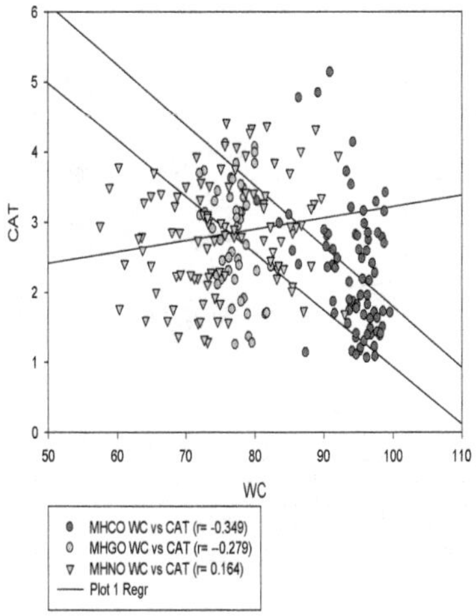

(g). GPx vs WC 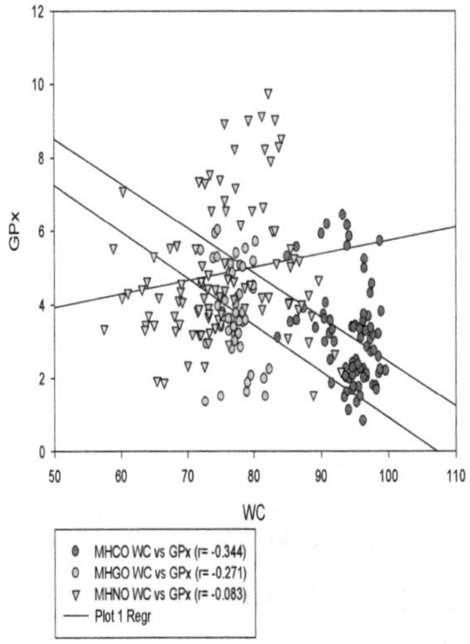 (h). FRAP vs WC

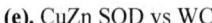

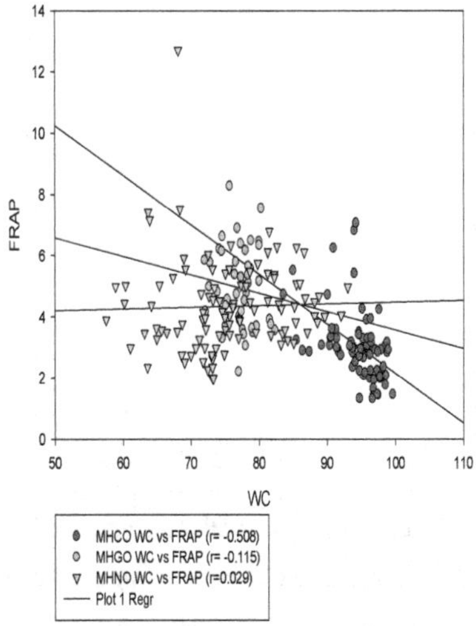

(i). CRP vs WC   (j). TNF alpha vs WC

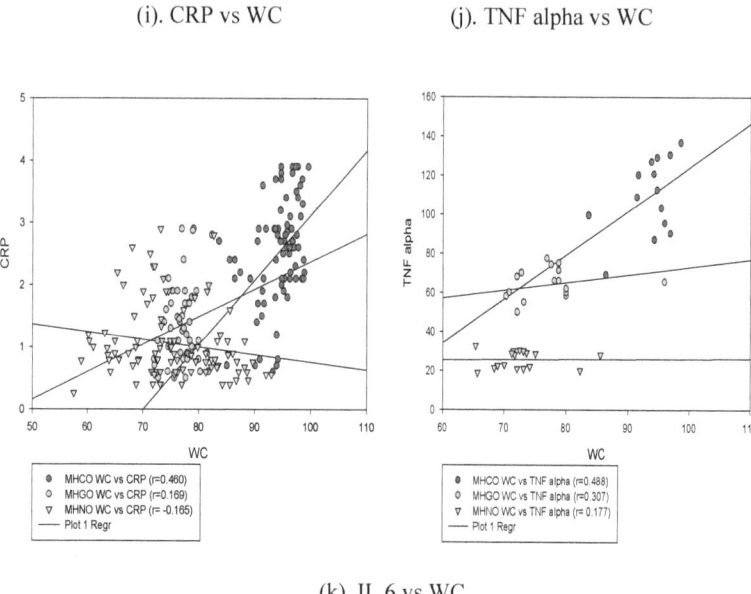

(k). IL 6 vs WC

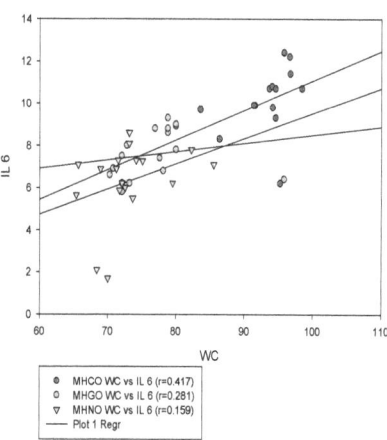

Figure 4.4.2: Correlation graphs for (a) OH Rad vs WC (b) FLOP vs WC (c) MDA vs WC, (d) PCO vs WC, (e) CuZn SOD vs WC, (f) CAT vs WC, (g) GPx vs WC, (h) FRAP vs WC, (i) CRP vs WC, (j) TNF alpha vs WC (k) IL 6 vs WC among MHNO, MHGO and MHCO respondents.

It is clear from the graphs that the OS and inflammatory markers do not correlate significantly with waist circumference in the MHNO respondents, the correlation is significant in the MHGO group but less striking than the highly significant correlation in the MHO group, indicating that central obesity has a more substantial impact on these indices than general obesity.

Discussion

In the present study, we compared the pattern of plasma/erythrocytic oxidative stress and inflammatory markers among metabolically healthy non-obese Controls (MHNO) and metabolically healthy adults with general and central obesity (MHGO and MHCO respectively). Our main finding reflects that there is a clear difference between MHGO and MHCO groups with regard to biochemical profile. Although selection criteria of obese group was absence of metabolic syndrome risk factors as prescribed by the NCEP: ATP III criteria, except obesity, there was a subtle difference in the patterns between MHCO and MHGO respondents. While MHGO respondents were more similar to MHNO Controls, MHCO respondents were at significantly higher risk for metabolic syndrome.

The MHGO respondents were also more similar to the MHNO Controls with regard to OS damage indices in plasma, including hydroxyl radicals, Plasma Fluorescent Oxidation Products (FLOP), and erythrocytic indices, namely MDA and PCO, while all of these indices were significantly higher in the (MHCO) Central Obesity group. The impact could be attributed to the difference in their antioxidant mechanisms, as erythrocytic enzymes, CuZn SOD, catalase, and plasma GPx, and total antioxidant capacity (TAC) were decreased in the MHCO respondents but not in the MHGO respondents, explaining their higher oxidative stress.

Hydroxyl radical, $^{\bullet}OH$, which is the neutral form of the hydroxide ion (OH^-) is a less studied index of free radical generation. Hydroxyl radicals are highly reactive (easily becoming hydroxyl groups) and consequently short-lived; produced from the decomposition of hydroperoxides (ROOH) and likely in Fenton chemistry, where trace amounts of reduced transition metals catalyze peroxide-mediated oxidations of organic compounds. The link between •OH and obesity has been reported by Li X et al [Li X, Fang P, Mai J et al., 2013]. In obese mice, lower vascular formation of ROS, including •OH has been reported, whereas the sensitivity to ROS is increased, suggesting a novel and important role of •OH in the regulation of vascular tone in disease status associated with increased body weight [Mundy AL, Haas E, Bhattacharya I et al., 2007]. In our study, •OH radical concentration was significantly higher than Controls in the centrally obese but the rise was not significant in the generally obese group who are more similar to non-obese Controls.

The findings are further validated by the estimation of fluorescent oxidation products (FLOPs), data on which is limited. FLOP assay are considered as a global measure of oxidation stress because they are generated from many different oxidation pathways [Jensen M K, Wang Y, Rimm EB et al. 2013; Wu T, Rifai N, Willett WC et al. 2007]. FLOP constitutes a stable and easily measured biomarker of cumulative metabolic and oxidative stress resulting from the interaction of reactive oxygen intermediates and free radicals with macromolecules and reflects oxidation products generated from several pathways including lipid, protein, DNA and carbohydrate oxidation [Fortner RT, Tworoger SS, Wu T et al. 2013]. Commonly used oxidation markers such as F2 – isoprostanes and malondialdehyde reflect only a part of oxidation, namely lipid oxidation. It has been suggested that FLOP assay is 10 -100 times more sensitive than measurement of malondialdehyde (MDA) estimated by the colorimetric thiobarbituric assay [Yoshida Y, Umeno A, Shichiri M et al. 2013].

The present study found that high levels of fluorescent oxidation products were more significantly associated with inflammatory and oxidative stress markers in central obesity (MHCO) group as compared to general obesity (MHGO) group, which indicated its potential to distinguish between central and general obesity. Plasma FLOP has been reported to independently predict the risk of subsequent coronary heart disease and other fatal and nonfatal cardiovascular disease events in epidemiologic studies [Wu T, Rifai N, Willett WC et al., 2007], but has not been investigated for possible differences with regard to fat distribution, which is observed in the present study.

Increase in lipid peroxidation of erythrocytic membrane and carbonylation of membrane protein are common consequences of systemic oxidative stress which are known to result from damage to the membrane in obesity [Brown LA, Kerr CJ, Whiting P et al., 2009; Tianying W, Rifai NL. Roberts II LJ et al., 2004; Yoshida Y, Umeno A, Shichiri M et al. 2013] as well as with various risk factors of metabolic syndrome [Furukawa S, Fujita T, Shimabukuro M et al., 2004]. Our results are supported by another study by Amirkhizi et al (2010) [Amirkhizi F, Siassi F, Djalali M et al., 2010] who have reported that abdominal obesity has been especially found to be associated with elevated oxidative stress and decreased total antioxidant capacity. Interestingly, there is evidence that the increased oxidative stress associated with obesity is reversible with weight loss and other interventions.

The overall pattern of oxidative stress measures, antioxidant enzymes and resultant total antioxidant capacity corroborate our earlier findings that homeostatic mechanisms operate to restore redox balance in lower stress states as compared to more severe redox aberrations [Singh S., Dwivedi A., Kumar S et al., 2019]. In this case, general obesity comes out as a milder stress state as compared to central obesity. Associations between oxidative stress markers and the inflammatory state in obesity have been reported, and the need to investigate the interplay between oxidative stress and inflammation to understand their cause-effect relationships with obesity [Iacobini C, Pugliese G, Fantauzzi FC et al. 2019].

The present study has also observed the trend of higher levels of inflammatory markers with higher oxidative stress in obese groups. The trend of lower impact on the MHGO group respondents as compared to the MHCO group respondents with regard to inflammatory markers, CRP, IL-6 and TNF-α is apparent.

When interrelationships of OS markers, antioxidant markers and inflammation were assessed with regard to BMI and waist circumference, the impact of WC was more than that of BMI in both general obesity as well as central obesity groups, again stressing the greater impact of central obesity.

The utility of anthropometric parameters to categorize individuals with different fat distribution has been a subject of recent investigations and links between risk factors of metabolic syndrome and central obesity have been highlighted [Lee JJ, Freeland-Graves JH, Pepper MR et al., 2014]. Significant difference in anthropometric indicators, inflammatory markers and estimated lifetime cardiovascular risk between the two adult obese subgroups differing in anthropometric measures has been reported [Khawaja KI, Mian SA, Fatima A et al., 2018]. A study on prepubescence showed the coexistence of increased obesity-related subclinical inflammation and decreased antioxidant capacity was observed which could predispose them to increased risk of long-term vascular damage [Vehapoglu A, Turkmen S, Goknar N et al., 2016] and there is evidence that anthropometric measures of central obesity are better predictors of cardiovascular disease (CVD) risk compared with general obesity measures in women [Goh LG, Dhaliwal SS, Welborn TA, et al., 2014]. Even normal-weight obese women whose body weight and BMI are normal but whose fat mass is >30%, have been reported to show early inflammatory status and oxidative stress patterns related to metabolic abnormalities occurring in obesity [Di Renzo L, Galvano F, Orlandi1 C et al., 2010], underlining the importance of fat mass over BMI as a risk factor for obesity related aberrations, with adiponectin being the proposed link between obesity and metabolic disturbance [Milewicz A, Jedrzejuk D, Dunajska K et al., 2010].

Adipose tissue has been reported to be responsible for inflammatory adipokines which in turn generate reactive oxygen species responsible for the high oxidative stress in obesity [Alkaabi J, Gariballa S, Sharma C et al., 2016], which has been especially attributed to visceral adipose tissue [Sánchez AF, Santillán EM, Bautista M et al., 2011]. These studies support the patterns observed in the present study.

The prevalence of metabolically healthy obese individuals is low, so a large number of potential individuals have to be screened for a large number of risk factors and other inclusion and exclusion criteria before a respondent can be found suitable for enrolment. Another limitation is the quantum of blood that any individual is comfortable in giving [Nijhawan LP, Janodia MD, Muddukrishna BS., et al., 2013]. The present study has tried to overcome these and has addressed issues related to redox balance and inflammatory markers in metabolically healthy individuals.

Further, since it is a cross-sectional study, hence it does not allow inferences regarding causality. However, the case-control design is efficient in controlling for confounding factors such as age and gender, which were matched; hence the design helped us in controlling for the confounding effect of BMI, allowing us to compare people with different fat distribution, as indexed by waist circumference, but the same BMI.

Chapter 4.5: To compare metabolically healthy obese (MHO) and metabolically unhealthy obese (MUHO) with metabolic syndrome respondents with regard to NCEP ATP III MetS risk factors, markers of oxidative stress, redox balance and inflammation.

The present chapter is designed to investigate the biochemical comparisons between metabolically healthy obese (MHO) and metabolically unhealthy obese (MUHO) respondents. As described in previous chapters, MHO is defined as absence of Metabolic Syndrome (MetS), as assessed by the NCEP ATP III prescribed criteria. Concomitant studies of these biochemical correlates were conducted in our lab on respondents suffering from obesity with MetS considered as metabolically unhealthy obesity (MUHO) by another investigator [http://hdl.handle.net/10603/283028], and it was desirable to assess the comparative biochemical study between metabolically healthy obesity (MHO) with metabolically unhealthy obesity (MUHO). MUHO comprised of obese respondents suffering from all five risk factors of MetS as prescribed by NCEP ATP III, and were designed as metabolically unhealthy obesity with metabolic syndrome (MUHO). They suffered from Central obesity, High Fasting plasma glucose, High Blood pressure (or treated for hypertension), Dyslipidemia (TG ≥ 150 mg/dl, HDL-C < 40 mg/dL (male) (DL), < 50 mg/dL (female).

The present study was conducted to compare biochemical measures in metabolically healthy obese (MHO) and metabolically unhealthy obesity (MUHO, obesity with metabolic syndrome). Respondents were matched for age. MHO and MUHO were matched for BMI (Table 4.5.1).

Table 4.5.1: General characteristics of respondents assigned to metabolically healthy obese (MHO) and metabolically unhealthy obese (MUHO) groups

Demographic Data	MHO	MUHO
N	102	102
Age (years)	55.3±13.8	59.0±8.8
Height (cm)	159.6±6.4	159.2±7.5
Weight (Kg)	82.8±6.4	83.4±8.1
Body Mass Index (Kg/m^2)	32.5±1.3	32.9±1.6

All values are expressed as Mean ± SD.

Table 4.5.2 represent NCEP ATP III prescribed diagnostic measures and other related clinical measures of respondents assigned to MHO and MUHO. Statistically significant differences (p<0.05) were also seen between MHO and MUHO with regard to waist circumference, fasting blood glucose, triglycerides, HDL-C, blood pressure, total cholesterol, LDL-cholesterol and cholesterol.

Table 4.5.2: NCEP ATP III prescribed diagnostic measures and other clinical biochemical measures of respondents assigned to metabolically healthy obese (MHO) and metabolically unhealthy obesity (MUHO)

	MHO	MUHO	P value
NCEP ATP III Diagnostic Criteria For Met S			
Waist circumference	101±11.9	113.2±3.9	<0.0001***
Fasting Blood Glucose	102.5±9.2	167.3±3.91	<0.0001***
Triglyceride	152.6±12.2	239.4±35.4	<0.0001***
HDL-Cholesterol	49±6.5	34.2±3.55	<0.0001***
Blood Pressure	122.5±4.9	148.9±12.0	<0.0001***
	80.9±4.8	95.3±9.5	<0.0001***
Other related biochemical measures			
Total Cholesterol	200 ±14.1	287.7±54.4	<0.0001***
Low density lipoprotein-C	120.6±16.9	175.4±31.8	<0.0001***

All values are expressed as Mean ± SD. Data were processed for t test analysis at p<0.05.

Figure 4.5.1 represents the relative percent difference of biochemical parameters between MHO and MUHO. Interestingly, the difference between MHO and MUHO for all the parameters except WC, SBP and DBP, was maximum for all pairs studied, indicating the greater the metabolic perturbations leads to the development of abnormality on MetS risk factors in MHO group respondents.

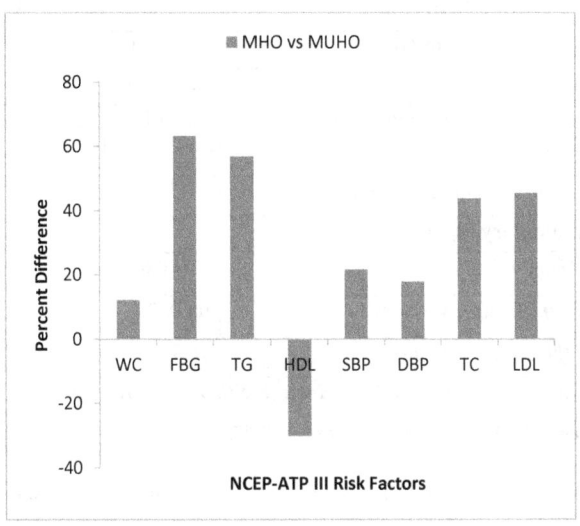

Figure 4.5.1: Relative per cent difference of NCEP ATP III diagnostic criteria for Met S, and related biochemical parameters between MHO and MUHO group.

Plasma/serum antioxidant markers GPx, FRAP, erythrocytic oxidative stress markers: MDA, PCO, CuZnSOD, catalase and circulating (serum) inflammatory markers: C-reactive protein (CRP), tumor necrosis factor alpha (TNF –α), interleukin 6 (IL- 6) were assessed in the groups and results are presented in Table 4.5.3.

Table 4.5.3: Erythrocytic and plasma oxidative stress markers of metabolically healthy obese (MHO) and metabolically unhealthy obesity (MUHO).

	MHO	MUHO	P value
Oxidative Stress Markers			
Erythrocytic MDA(nmoles/g Hb)	3.47±1.1	5.53±1.2	<0.0001***
Erythrocytic PCO(nmole/g Hb)	2.55±0.8	4.53±1.3	<0.0001***
Erythrocytic CuZnSOD(unit /g Hb)	2.84±1.1	1.21±0.7	<0.0001***
Erythrocytic CAT(unit/g Hb)	2.29±0.6	1.01±0.6	<0.0001***
Plasma GPx (nmole/min/mg plasma protein)	4.3±1.8	1.68±1.6	<0.0001***
FRAP (µmole/ml of plasma)	2.97±0.9	1.40±0.9	<0.0001***
Inflammatory Markers			
CRP (mg/ml)	1.5±0.8	3.19±0.7	<0.0001***
TNF –α (N=30+28) (pg/ml)	95.0±32	275.7±42.9	<0.0001***
IL 6 (N=24+28) (pg/ml)	16.7±6.7	48.8±10.8	<0.0001***

All values are expressed as Mean ± SD. Data were processed for t test analysis followed by Mann Whitney test at p<0.05.

(MDA: Malondialdehyde, PCO: Protein carbonyl, SOD: Superoxide dismutase, FRAP: Ferric reducing ability of plasma, GPX: Glutathione Peroxidase, CAT: Catalase, CRP: C reactive protein, TNF–α: Tumor necrosis factor alpha, IL 6: Interleukin 6)

All OS indices, MDA, PCO, CuZn SOD, catalase, and plasma GPx, TAC as FRAP and inflammatory markers CRP, TNF alpha and IL 6 showed significant difference between MHO and MUO. Since all the biochemical markers showed significant difference, the percent difference was calculated between MHO and MUHO group respondents and is presented in Fig 4.5.2. Maximum difference was found for PCO followed by MDA while antioxidant markers showed different pattern from MDA and PCO. There was a consistent decline in CuZn SOD, CAT, GPx and FRAP parameters. Since all are the indices of antioxidant capacity and their decrease and increase in OS markers MDA, PCO is responsible for transient phase transmission from MHO to MUHO.

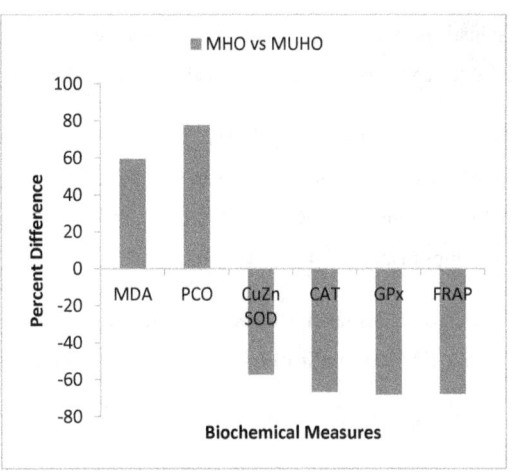

Figure 4.5.2: Relative per cent difference in oxidative stress markers between MHO and MUHO experimental groups.

The percent differences for the groups under investigation is assessed for inflammatory markers, CRP, TNF alpha, IL 6 and is presented in Fig 4.5.3. We have found similar patterns as MDA and PCO. Maximum percent change was found for TNF alpha followed by IL 6 and CRP.

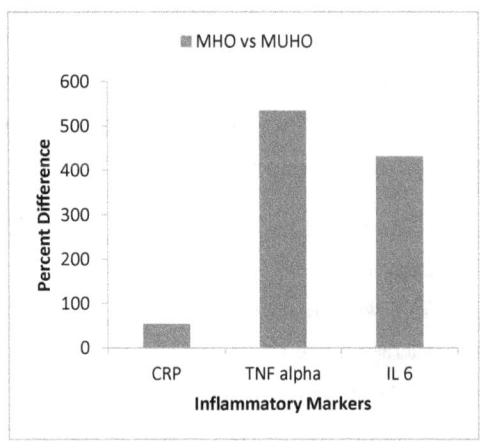

Figure: 4.5.3 Relative per cent difference in inflammatory markers CRP, TNF alpha and IL 6 MHO and MUHO.

Further statistical tools were employed to explore whether this had some functional significance for comparing the biochemical impacts of these two conditions.

Since BMI >30 for MHO and MUHO was the confounding variable thus waist circumference used as independent variable to find out correlation coefficients between WC with indices of OS and inflammatory markers were obtained to assess interrelationships (Table 4.5.4).

Table 4.5.4: Interrelationships between oxidative stress (OS) markers with waist circumference (WC), as indicated by Pearson's correlation coefficientsr.

		MDA	PCO	SOD	CAT	GPx	FRAP	CRP	TNF alpha	IL 6
WC	MHO	0.294*	0.281*	-0.176	-0.194	-0.217	-0.245*	0.234	0.321*	0.160
	MUO	0.416*	0.357*	-0.256*	-0.245*	-0.268*	-0.341*	0.319*	0.626*	0.352*

indicates statistical significance at p<0.05.

Oxidative stress markers MDA and PCO and inflammatory markers CRP, TNF alpha and IL 6 showed significantly strong correlation with WC in MUHO but reverse pattern was found for antioxidant markers CuZn SOD, CAT, GPx and FRAP. MHO group respondents showed significant positive correlation with WC with regard to MDA, PCO and for TNF alpha but none of the antioxidant markers except FRAP showed any relationship with WC. Since these are required for ameliorating OS and bringing the system back to equilibrium.

Hence, oxidative stress markers were further assessed for their role as relative risk factors for distinguishing between metabolically unhealthy obesity with metabolic syndrome (MUHO) with metabolically healthy obesity (MHO). Area under receiver operating characteristic curve (AUC) were calculated for MDA, PCO, CuZn SOD, CAT, GPx and FRAP, as shown in figure 4.5.4 (a-f).

Fig 4.5.4 (a). MDA (MHO Vs MUHO) **(b).** PCO (MHO Vs MUHO)

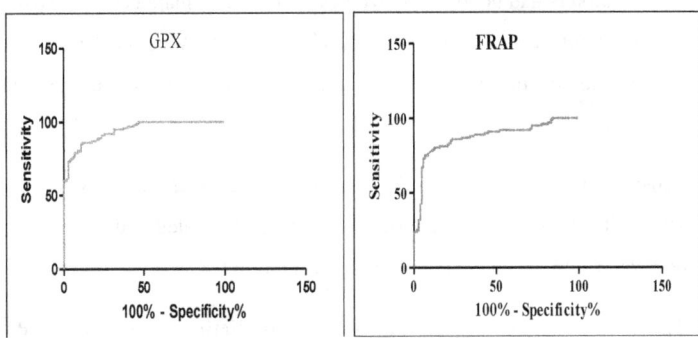

(c). CuZn SOD (MHO Vs MUHO) **(d)** CAT (MHO vs MUHO)

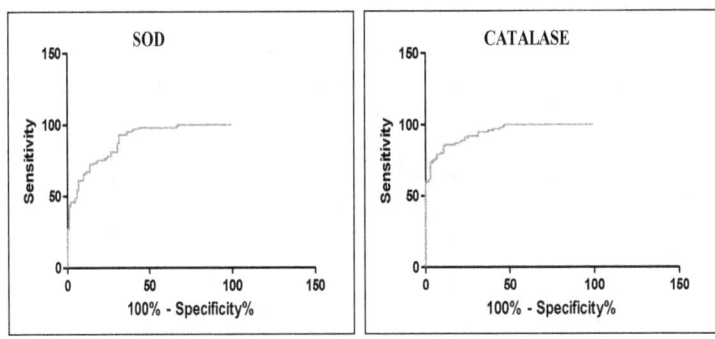

(e). GPx (MHO vs MUHO) **(f).** FRAP (MHO vs MUHO)

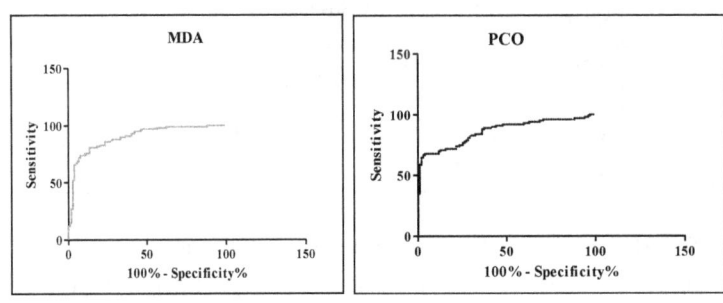

Figure 4.5.4 Area under receiver operating characteristic curve (AUC) for oxidative stress markers (a) MDA, (b) PCO, (c), CuZn SOD, (d) CAT, (e) GPx and (f) FRAP.

The graphical representation of the AUC curve for all OS markers indicated that all the biomarkers had good predictive power to discriminate between MHO and MUHO because their AUC curve was very close to y axis corner (AUC > 0.85). These markers indicating high clinical utility due to high values of specificity and sensitivity.

Table 4.5.5 represent the AUC values at 95 % confidence interval of sensitivity and specificity through which cut off points were calculated and by using these cut offs odds ratio were calculated between MHO and MUHO.

Table 4.5.5: AUC of OS indices for predicting their use in distinguishing metabolically unhealthy obesity with metabolic syndrome (MUHO) and metabolically healthy obesity (MHO).

	GROUPS	AUC	SE	95% CI (AUC)	P VALUE	Cut off	Odds ratio (OR)	95% CI (OR)
MDA	MHO vs. MUHO	0.896	0.022	0.852-0.94	<0.0001	>3.6	23.8	68.7, 62.2
PCO	MHO vs. MUHO	0.862	0.02	0.81-0.91	<0.0001	>2.1	8.8	3.26, 23.6
CuZn SOD	MHO vs. MUHO	0.88	0.022	0.841-0.928	<0.0001	<1.7	15	7.52, 29.9
CAT	MHO vs. MUHO	0.9	0.02	0.86-0.92	<0.0001	<1.2	54.8	19.8, 151.5
GPx	MHO vs. MUHO	0.94	0.01	0.91-0.91	<0.0001	<3.4	13.1	6.33, 27.01
FRAP	MHO vs. MUHO	0.872	0.02	0.82-0.92	<0.0001	<1.1	88.5	11.8, 659.9

The AUC values usually range from 0.5 (no discriminant capacity) to 1.0 (Perfect Discriminant Capacity). All OS indices studies here (MDA, PCO, CuZn SOD, CAT, GPx and FRAP) had high AUC values (AUC >0.86), hence all these markers have good distinguishing capacity to differentiate MHO and MUHO group. The antioxidant markers CuZn SOD, CAT, GPx and FRAP appear to be good clinical markers with high AUC values. Odds ratio (ORs) obtained from cut off value describe associations of biomarkers with clinical status, hence these were also computed. There was an 88.5 times probability that FRAP would be lower than the cut-off of 1.1 in the ObMetS respondents than those who were obese without symptoms of metabolic syndrome. FRAP was followed by lower erythrocytic catalase (54.8), higher MDA (23.8), lower erythrocytic SOD (15) and plasma GPx (13.10) and higher PCO (8.8).

Discussion

Previous chapters described different aspects of metabolically healthy obesity (MHO) in terms of BMI, age, gender, body fat distribution, assessed by waist circumference. Metabolically healthy obesity is a unique phenotype of obesity without significant metabolic perturbations, while metabolically unhealthy obesity (MUHO) is defined to include respondents who suffer from all risk factors of metabolic syndrome.

As expected, the MUHO group had statistically significant and greater aberration for all the parameters with regard to NCEP ATP III risk factors for MetS, even as some departure from normal was also observed in the MHO. Percent difference between MUHO and MHO was maximum for fasting plasma glucose (FPG), an index marker of hyperglycemia, followed by triglyceride (TG) and high density lipoprotein (HDL), index markers of dyslipidemia, indicating that they may be important MetS risk factors predisposing conversion of MHO to MUHO. This is supported by studies which observe that metabolically healthy obesity phenotype (MHO) represents favorable metabolic profile in contrast to metabolically unhealthy obesity (MUHO), despite the similar amount of body fat [Singh S., Dwivedi A., Kumar S., Mittal PC., 2019; http://hdl.handle.net/10603/283028; Eckel N, Li Y, Kuxhaus O, et al., 2018]. A previous cohort study conducted on Chinese population has shown that metabolically healthy obesity (MHO) was a transient stage which lies between metabolically healthy normal weight (MHN) and metabolically unhealthy overweight/obesity (MUOO) and MHO was associated with increased risk of coronary artery diseases and heart failure. [Gao M, Lv J, Yu C, et al., 2020]. However, it is presently unclear whether individuals of MHO phenotype will move towards metabolically unhealthy profile with time hence we need to understand the underlying metabolic regulatory mechanism in development of MHO to MUHO and how to prevent it with lifestyle modifications.

The results further suggested the maximum systemic oxidative damage in MUHO group compared to MHO as indexed by OS and antioxidant markers. It was found that free radical induced oxidative damage in lipid and protein moieties in the erythrocytic membrane, indicated by significantly higher level of MDA and PCO in MUHO group as compared to MHO, indicating the greater disturbance in homeostatic redox status in MUHO as distinct from MHO. The antioxidant enzymes CuZn SOD, CAT, GPx and total antioxidant capacity (TAC) in terms of FRAP showed significant decrease compared with their MHO counterparts as expected, and reported by us earlier [Singh S., Dwivedi A., Kumar S., Mittal PC., 2019]. Studies comparing healthy and unhealthy obesity are missing, but recently, our findings are supported by a recent study conducted by Lejawa et al [Lejawa, M., Osadnik, K., Osadnik, T, et al., 2021] who observed total oxidation status (TOS), total antioxidant capacity was significantly correlated with relative telomere length (r TL) in metabolically unhealthy obesity with MetS abnormalities. Telomere shortens in MUO respondents related to metabolic dysregulation and increased oxidative stress while telomere length was not influenced by obesity itself in MHO respondents. Further Lejawa et al suggested that telomere length plays an important role in pathogenesis of metabolic syndrome in metabolically healthy obesity.

Florinela et al [FlorinelaCˇatoi, A.,Elena Pârvu A., Andreicut, AD, et al., 2018] did not find significant difference regarding total oxidant status (TOS) and total antioxidant response (TAR) between metabolically healthy morbid obese (MHNO) and metabolically unhealthy morbid obese with metabolic syndrome (MUHMO) while nitrite and nitrate oxide (NOx) was significantly higher in MUHMO. The results of our work suggest that metabolically unhealthy obesity is linked with metabolic abnormalities and anthropometric indices such as BMI and waist circumference are closely linked with oxidative stress markers: MDA, PCO which are inversely correlated with antioxidant enzymes CuZn SOD, CAT, GPx and FRAP.

Still, there is lack of data whether metabolic abnormalities linked to MUHO increases the degree of underlying redox imbalance or whether early manifestation of redox imbalance in the pathophysiology of metabolic syndrome linked to obesity rather than a consequence.

Obesity is associated with low grade chronic inflammation [Das UN., 2001]. Inflammatory markers CRP, TNF alpha, IL 6 and other cytokines and adipokines are linked with metabolic perturbations. These inflammatory markers such as CRP, TNF-α and IL-6 are known to be secreted from adipose tissue and were found to be significantly higher in metabolically unhealthy obesity (MUHO) to their MHO counterparts. Further all these parameters were significantly positively correlated with BMI. In a similar study conducted on Brazilian population [Shaharyar S., Roberson LL., Jamal O., 2015], it was found that hs-CRP was found to be highest in metabolically unhealthy overweight/obesity as compared to other groups studied. Epidemiological evidence has demonstrated that normal adipose tissue function has been associated to healthier metabolic profile even in obese phenotypes [Bluher M., 2010]. Adipose tissue is highly dynamic endocrine gland responsible for production of a large number of adipocytokines. It has been reported that these adipocytokines are responsible for metabolic health status associated with obesity. The MHO phenotypes represent reduced inflammatory profile which provides unique protective mechanisms in these individuals but as body fat increases, these adipocytokines uncouple the inflammatory signal transduction which causes metabolic health transition of MHO to MUHO [Alam I., Pin Ng T., Larbi A., 2012].

It has been reported that biomarkers are used as diagnostic tool and used in treatment of wide range of diseases. AUC analysis is the best statistical tool to measure the predictive value of various biomarkers. [El-Ansary A, Bjørklund G., Chirumbolo S., et al., 2017]. The OS markers were further analyzed as individual risk factors to distinguish MHO from MUHO, by obtaining area under curve (AUC) to calculate cut off values through which odds ratio were calculated. Although OS markers studied here had high clinical utility but FRAP emerged as the best diagnostic biomarker for assessing MUHO. There was an 88.5 times probability that FRAP would be lower for unhealthy obese respondents having metabolic syndrome than for respondents who were representing healthier metabolic profile without any metabolic complications referred as MHO. The odds of having a lower erythrocytic catalase were 54.8 times, a higher MDA 23.8 times, a lower erythrocytic SOD 15 times, plasma GPx 13 times and higher PCO 8.8 times. Thus, our study indicates that FRAP is the best candidate to qualify as a biomarker to distinguish between MUHO and MHO, followed by erythrocytic catalase, SOD, GPx and PCO in that order, which are also candidates of diagnostic significance.

From the above, we can conclude that the redox balance is most severely disturbed in the group suffering from MUHO. The strikingly high increase in FRAP makes it a useful candidate for study of homeostatic balance in metabolic syndrome which may be seen as a breakdown of the homeostatic processes which depend on a large number of enzymes such as SOD, catalase, GPx etc. and also on non-enzymatic antioxidants. Thus, FRAP can be proposed as an important diagnostic tool for prognosis in MUHO respondents and more in-depth studies are suggested in this direction.

Based on the foregoing, we can conclude that the redox homeostasis is significantly more disturbed in the metabolically unhealthy obesity with metabolic syndrome (MUHO) as compared to metabolically healthy obesity (MHO).

SUMMARY AND CONCLUSION

The importance of maintenance of body weight in humans throughout adult life to promote good health is being increasingly recognized. While body weight can be both lower and higher than normal, overweight/obesity has attracted more attention, and is considered to be one of the most challenging health risks of present time. The main etiological factor of obesity is energy imbalance between energy intake and expenditure due to reduced physical activity. The Body mass index (BMI) is the most accepted obesity index marker according to World Health Organization (WHO), to define obesity into different grades, which is calculated by dividing the weight in kilograms by the square of the height in meters (m^2). WHO categorizes obesity in adults into different grades, those with BMI$\leq$25 kg/m^2 as non-obese; 25-30 kg/m^2 as overweight, and BMI$\geq$30 kg/m^2 as obese

The last few decades have seen a rapid rise in research linking increase in body weight to several adverse effects on health, such as predisposition to many diseases such as diabetes, hypertension, chronic heart diseases, osteoarthritis, cancer, and consequent reduced life expectancy.

However, not all obese people exhibit metabolic complications and a distinct phenotype of obese individuals without occurrence of metabolic complications known as metabolically healthy obesity (MHO) has been reported. Most weight management studies are related to an unhealthy metabolic profile of obesity and meaningful data linked to metabolically healthy obesity (MHO) is lacking. Such studies are important because such individuals continue to show a good biochemical profile, although some reports suggest that MHO may be converted to metabolically unhealthy obesity over time or as age advances. A greater understanding of the MHO individual has important implications for therapeutic decision making, the characterization of subjects in research protocols and medical education.

Excess adipose tissue in metabolically unhealthy obesity causes systemic oxidative stress which leads to development of oxidative damage, triggering irregular production of adipokines and inflammatory markers. Oxidative stress can be measured by many oxidative damage indices and its amelioration can be measured by a set of enzymatic and non-enzymatic antioxidants. The overall impact is even more complex to measure. Any *in vivo* biochemical system works to reach equilibrium, and redox balance is an important outcome, the measurement of which can give an estimate of the overall homeostatic balance achieved.

In view of the foregoing, the present investigation was undertaken to study the metabolically healthy overweight and obesity phenotype that have a healthy biochemical profile. They do not display the NCEP ATP III risk factors for metabolic syndrome. Since obesity associated with these metabolic aberrations has been found to be linked to increased oxidative stress and inflammatory biomarkers and a disturbed redox balance, these parameters were assessed in metabolically healthy overweight and obese groups, and compared with their non-obese counterparts.

Oxidative stress indices employed to assess the damage caused by free radicals were hydroxyl radicals (OH Radicals), Fluorescent oxidation products (FLOP) which are direct indicators of oxidative stress, Malondialdehyde (MDA) for erythrocytic lipid peroxidation and protein carbonyls (PCO) for erythrocytic protein carbonylation. The levels of these are modulated by the antioxidant enzymes, which include superoxide dismutase (CuZn SOD), catalase (CAT), and glutathione peroxidase (GPx). The overall prooxidant-antioxidant balance of any biological system depends on balance between the large number of antioxidant mediated biological processes which include many enzymes and an even larger number of non-enzymatic antioxidants such as vitamins and other free radical scavengers. It is not possible to measure all the OS markers nor is it easy to evaluate so much data, hence it is important to estimate total antioxidant capacity (TAC). This has been done here in terms of ferric reducing ability of plasma (FRAP) which measures non-enzymatic antioxidant capacity. It is a commonly used index marker of non-enzymatic total antioxidant capacity in plasma, but it is known to be also affected by the enzymes in the milieu, and its decline indicates poor redox balance.

The OS induced inflammation plays a significant role in obesity associated pathogenesis. Tumor necrosis factor alpha (TNF alpha), interleukin 6 (IL 6) and C reactive protein (CRP) were also measured in this study because TNF alpha is an important proinflammatory marker secreted by adipose tissue which induces secretion of the other proinflammatory markers, IL6 and CRP.

To study the effect of obesity indices on oxidative stress markers, antioxidant balance and inflammatory markers, we have adopted the case control design which are observational, no intervention is attempted and no attempt is made to alter the course of the disease. The goal is to retrospectively determine the exposure to the risk factor of interest from each of the two groups of individuals: cases and controls.

For this study, the human model was selected for better understanding of a realistic in vivo scenario to assess the relationship among obesity indices, namely, BMI and waist circumference, OS and inflammatory markers. Consequently, the present investigation was undertaken to study Indian metabolically healthy adults aged 20 to 80 years in order to assess the impact of their obesity indices on selected biochemical markers of NCEP ATP III prescribed risk factors for Met S, oxidative stress, redox balance, and inflammation with regard to BMI, age, gender, body fat distribution and metabolic health.

In chapter 4.1, a comparison was made among metabolically healthy (MH) non obese controls, overweight and obese respondents with regard to markers of NCEP ATP III Met S risk factors and markers of oxidative stress, redox balance and inflammation.

In section A of this chapter, we compared NCEP ATP Met S risk factors, oxidative stress and inflammatory markers among metabolically healthy (MH) non obese controls, overweight and obese respondents, grouped as per WHO guidelines. As expected, within the metabolically healthy (MH) respondents, BMI significantly impacted the NCEP ATP III prescribed norms. Though all groups are selected only if the metabolic stress related risk factors fall within normal range, the MH non obese controls (MHNO) group had the healthiest profile, followed by the overweight (MHOw) group while the obese (MHO) group had the maximum aberration. Differences were minimum between the MH non obese controls (MHNO) and MH overweight (MHOw) respondents, but were significant between overweight (MHOw) and obese (MHO).

With regard to OS indices, all groups differ with regard to all oxidative stress indicators, antioxidant enzymes and inflammatory markers. However, it was interesting that differences between MH non obese controls and MH overweight groups with regard to most parameters were minimal compared to those between MH overweight (MHOw) and MH obese (MHO) groups. Inflammatory markers, CRP, TNF-alpha and IL-6 in all groups were significantly correlated to BMI.

The findings also support previous findings from our lab that the homeostatic mechanism in obesity with MetS depends on antioxidant enzymes, CuZn SOD, catalase (CAT) and Glutathione peroxidase (GPx) which consequently modulate levels of oxidative stress markers, malondialdehyde (MDA) and protein carbonylation (PCO) and total antioxidant capacity. When these enzymes decrease, the entire system moves towards increased oxidative stress, and in some cases of mild disturbance, the overall oxidative stress is not visibly increased due to the ability of the system to restore equilibrium. The same pattern is observed in the present study. Results indicate breakdown of this adaptation in the metabolically healthy obese (MHO) but not in the metabolically healthy overweight (MHOw) which are more like the MH non obese controls than the obese (MHO).

In section B, we have compared **two BMI classification guidelines** with regard to **NCEP ATP III Met S risk factors, oxidative stress and inflammatory markers among metabolically healthy (MH) non obese controls, overweight and obese respondents.** Some researchers have indicated the need for ethnic specific norms to formulate overweight and obese categories based on BMI. While the WHO norms have been adopted worldwide, Asian guidelines have been promulgated which subdivide the WHO defined non-obese into two groups, the non-obese and the overweight, to accommodate the specific ethnic characteristics of Indians. When we did this, no major significant difference was found between the two subgroups of the Asian guidelines, nor between either of these groups with the WHO defined non-obese group. We can conclude that, for metabolically healthy respondents, our data does not indicate any justification for regrouping the obesity criteria with regard to the Asian Guidelines for their ethnicity. Hence in all subsequent chapters, we have employed the WHO criteria for grouping our respondents into normal weight, overweight and obese.

Oxidative stress and its consequences on metabolic diseases is known to be age-dependent.

Hence, In chapter 4.2, metabolically healthy non obese controls (MHNO), metabolically healthy overweight (MHOw) and metabolically healthy obese (MHO) respondents were compared with regard to markers of oxidative stress, redox balance and inflammation in relation to age. The respondents of the three study groups MHNO, MHOw and MHO, aged 20-80 years were divided into three age groups, Young Adults (YA, 20-39 years), Middle-aged Adults (MA, 40-59 years), and Elderly (EA, >60 years). All the groups of metabolically healthy respondents: non-obese, overweight and obese showed a significant positive correlation between body weight and BMI in all age groups from 20 to 60+ years. Despite having NCEP-ATP risk factor values within prescribed range, metabolically healthy non-obese controls (MHNO) had healthier metabolic profiles at all ages, the obese began with a relatively unhealthier profile but it did not worsen with age while the metabolically healthy overweight began with a healthy profile but as they aged, it moved to an unhealthier profile.

OS indices were selected to assess redox homeostasis, with serum OH radicals and FLOP, erythrocytic MDA and PCO as indices of oxidative stress, antioxidant enzymes, erythrocytic Cu-Zn SOD, Catalase and plasma GPx, and total antioxidant capacity FRAP. These parameters were instrumental in suggesting that antioxidant enzymes did not get disrupted with age in the metabolically healthy normal weight controls (MHNO) who maintained efficient homeostasis through all ages, but in both, overweight (MHOw) and obese (MHO) groups, age-wise changes show increase in oxidative stress. This was marginal in the overweight (MHOw) group but worsened in the obese (MHO). A similar pattern of worsening with age is evident in the inflammatory markers in the metabolically healthy overweight (MHOw) and obese (MHO) groups but no age-related change is evident in the MH non obese controls.

Gender differences are known to exist in incidence of metabolic diseases, but has not attracted the attention it deserves. Therefore the data was evaluated to explore for possible gender differences.

In chapter 4.3, the gender-specific association of NCEP ATP III MetS risk factors, oxidative stress, redox balance and inflammatory markers on metabolically healthy non obese controls (MHNO), overweight (MHOw) and obese (MHO) respondents were studied. Gender is a crucial determinant of obesity as well as oxidative stress. The study groups described in Chapter 4.1 were analyzed for gender differences and the findings are presented in this chapter. There is no gender difference between metabolically healthy normal weight (MHNO) and overweight (MHOw) males and females but the obese (MHO) group females had higher values of triglyceride (TG), total cholesterol (TC), low density lipoproteins (LDL), fasting blood glucose levels and waist circumference than males. The main gender difference in redox state was that metabolically healthy non obese controls (MHNO) and overweight (MHOw) respondents did not show any significant modification in pattern. In their obese (MHO) counterparts, however, all OS indices were higher in females, but they also had a higher level of antioxidant enzymes, and consequently a higher total antioxidant capacity. This was an important finding because it indicated better adaptation and restoration of homeostasis in the obese (MHO) females. Similarly, no major gender difference was apparent with regard to the inflammatory markers studied in the MH non obese controls (MHNO) and overweight (MHOw) phenotypes, but in the obese (MHO) groups, females had higher TNF $-\alpha$ and, to some extent IL6 also. None of the parameters showed any significant gender difference with increasing BMI in the MH non obese controls, while males but not females of the metabolically healthy overweight (MHOw) phenotype were affected, but, in the obese (MHO) phenotype, the overall pattern was similar in the males and females, showing a significant dependence on BMI with significant increase in all OS indices and decline in antioxidant enzymes and consequent decline in FRAP with BMI.

Distribution of body fat is also an important determinant of the biochemical consequences of obesity, especially that which is linked to metabolic syndrome. Central obesity, defined as a high abdominal girth, is more detrimental than general obesity characterized by a high body mass index in metabolically unhealthy obese. Whether this is also a pattern in the metabolically healthy groups is an important question, which was addressed in the next chapter.

In chapter 4.4, comparisons were made among metabolically healthy (MH) non obese controls (MHNO), and those with general obesity (MHGO) or central obesity (MHCO) with regard to the NCEP ATP III risk factors, markers of oxidative stress, redox balance and inflammation. In all the groups of metabolically healthy respondents, MHNO, MHGO and MHCO group respondents, WC significantly impacts the NCEP-ATP III risk factors of metabolic syndrome. Although, all the risk factors in all groups fell within normal range, as designed by the inclusion criteria, maximum aberration was found in MHCO group followed by MHGO group while metabolically healthy non obese controls (MHNO) represented the healthiest metabolic profile.

OS indices were measured to assess the redox balance. The MHGO respondents were also more similar to the MHNO with regard to OS damage indices in plasma, including hydroxyl radicals, Plasma Fluorescent Oxidation Products (FLOP), and erythrocytic indices, namely MDA and PCO, while all of these indices were significantly higher in the Central Obesity (MHCO) group. The impact could be attributed to the difference in their antioxidant mechanisms, as erythrocytic enzymes, CuZn SOD, catalase, and plasma GPx, and total antioxidant capacity (FRAP) were decreased in the MHCO group respondents but not in the MHGO respondents, explaining their higher oxidative stress. Inflammatory markers CRP, TNF-alpha and IL 6 were significantly correlated to WC in MHCO and MHGO group while no significant correlation was found in MHNO group respondents.

It is important to compare the metabolically healthy obese with their metabolically unhealthy counterparts. Hence, data from a group of respondents having severe MetS, also from our lab was compared with the present metabolically healthy obese group.

In chapter 4.5, a comparison was made between metabolically healthy obese (MHO) and metabolically unhealthy obese (MUO) respondents with regard to markers of oxidative stress, redox balance and inflammation. The MHO was selected to have NCEP ATP III risk factors within prescribed range and represented the healthy metabolic profile while the MUHO group had all five risk factors of MetS as prescribed by NCEP ATP III, and were designed as metabolically unhealthy obese.

Both groups differed with regard to all oxidative stress indicators, antioxidant enzymes and inflammatory markers. Free radical induced damage particularly in lipids measured in terms of malondialdehyde (MDA), and damage in proteins measured in terms of protein carbonylation (PCO) and inflammatory markers CRP, TNF alpha, IL6 was higher in MUHO group than in MHO group and can be good markers to distinguish between healthy and unhealthy obesity. The level of antioxidant enzymes, CuZn SOD, CAT, GPx and total antioxidant capacity in terms of FRAP were lower in MUHO group than in MHO, indicating the greater disturbance in the homeostatic processes in MUHO, as distinct from MHO. A lower total antioxidant capacity as indexed by FRAP showed the highest Odds Ratio, indicating that it was the best index to distinguish unhealthy and healthy obese groups, followed by lower erythrocytic catalase, higher MDA, lower erythrocytic SOD and plasma GPx and higher PCO.

Thus, the present investigations were centered on comparisons of metabolically healthy normal weight, overweight and obese groups. They were designated as metabolically healthy because they did not test positive for any of the NCEP ATP III prescribed norms. The main findings that emerge are:

1. Some aberrations in the NCEP ATP III norms were observed in metabolically healthy overweight and obese which correlated with body mass index and waist circumference.
2. The overweight group was closer metabolically as well as with regard to redox balance to the non-obese counterparts than to the obese group.
3. The redox balance was disturbed in the metabolically healthy obese, who had higher erythrocytic oxidative stress damage as indexed by higher levels of OS

indices, namely hydroxyl radicals, Fluorescent Oxidation Products (FLOP), malondialdehyde, mainly due to a decline in the erythrocytic antioxidant enzymes, super oxide dismutase and catalase, and, in most cases, it also reflects in plasma GPx, leading to a decline in overall antioxidant status. However, this pattern was not found in the overweight counterparts, where the antioxidant enzymes were higher and the decline in overall antioxidant status was not evident, indicating homeostatic redox balance.

4. This reaffirms earlier findings from our lab that the more severe aberrations result in greater decline in these enzymes which is reflected in a decline in the FRAP value. Since, FRAP is an index of non-enzymatic total antioxidant capacity, it is suggested that the entire systemic milieu is interconnected and the overall homeostatic processes are linked.

5. The milder aberrations as represented by the metabolically healthy overweight group display a redox profile which is indicative of adaptation mediated through modulations in the antioxidant enzymes.

6. The adaptive response leading to a better redox balance is more in the younger age groups and in the overweight females as compared to the older age groups and overweight male counterparts. The gender difference is not sustained in the more severe obese group.

7. The metabolically healthy overweight groups are at low risk to develop metabolically unhealthy biochemical profiles, but the metabolically healthy obese are more likely to develop unhealthy biochemical profiles.

REFERENCES

1. Ahima RS. (2009). Connecting obesity, aging and diabetes. Nat Med. 15, 996–997.
2. Ahirwar R. and Mondal PR. (2019). Prevalence of obesity in India: A systematic review. Diabetes & Metabolic Syndrome: Clinical Research & Reviews. 13, 318-321.
3. Alam I, Pin Ng T, Larbi A. (2012). Does Inflammation Determine Whether Obesity Is Metabolically Healthy or Unhealthy? The Aging Perspective Mediators of Inflammation Article ID 456456, doi:10.1155/2012/456456.
4. Alberti KG and Zimmet PZ. (1998). Definition, diagnosis and classification of diabetes mellitus and its complications. Part1 diagnosis and classification of diabetes mellitus provisional report of a WHO consultation, Diabet Med, 15:539–53.
5. Alkaabi J, Gariballa S, Sharma C et al. (2016). Inflammatory markers and cardiovascular risks among overweight-obese Emirati women. BMC Res Notes. 9:355.
6. Amirkhizi F, Siassi F, Djalali M et al., 2010 Evaluation of oxidative stress and total antioxidant capacity in women with general and abdominal adiposity. Obesity Research & Clinical Practice2010; 4, e209—e216
7. Amirkhizi F, Siassi F, Minaie S et al. (2007). Is obesity associated with increased plasma lipid peroxidation and oxidative stress in women? ARYA Atheroscler J, 2(4):189–92.
8. Arterburn DE, Crane PK, Sullivan SD. (2004). The coming epidemic of obesity in elderly Americans. Journal of the American Geriatrics Society. 52 (11):1907–1912.
9. Balistreri CR, Caruso C, Candore G. (2010). The role of adipose tissue and adipokines in obesity-related inflammatory diseases. MediatInflamm. 2010:802078.
10. Barp J, Araujo AS, Fernandes TR et al. (2002). Myocardial antioxidant and

oxidative stress changes due to sex hormones. Braz J Med Biol Res. 35: 1075–81.

11. Beigh SH and Jain S. (2012). Prevalence of metabolic syndrome and gender differences. Bioinformation, 8(13):613–616.

12. Beneditti A, Comporti M, Fulceri R. et al. (1984). Cytotoxic aldehydes originating from the peroxidation of liver microsomal lipids. Identification of 4, 5 dihydroxydecenal. Biochem. Biophys. Acta. 792: 172-181.

13. Benzie IF and Strain JJ. (1996). The ferric reducing ability of plasma as a measure of antioxidant power: the FRAP assay. Anal Biochem, 239 (1):70-6.

14. BhansaliS, Bhansali A, Dhawan V. (2017). Favourable metabolic profile sustains mitophagy and prevents metabolic abnormalities in metabolically healthy obese individuals. Diabetology& Metabolic Syndrome. 9:99. 24.

15. Bluher M. (2010). The distinction of metabolically 'healthy' from 'unhealthy' obese individuals. CurrOpinLipidol. 21:38-43.

16. Blum J., and Fridovich, I. (1985). Inactivation of glutathione peroxidise by superoxide radicals. Arch. Biochem. Biophys. 240: 500-508

17. BondiaPons I, Ryan L, Martinez J A. (2012). Oxidative stress and inflammation interactions in human obesity. J PhysiolBiochem. 68:701–711.

18. Bournat JC and Brown CW. (2010). Mitochondrial dysfunction in obesity. Current Opinion in Endocrinology, Diabetes, and Obesity. 17: 446–452.

19. Bravata DM, Wells CK, Concato J et al. (2004). Two measures of insulin sensitivity provided similar information in a U.S. population. Journal of Clinical Epidemiology, 57(11):1214–1217.

20. Brown LA, Kerr CJ, Whiting P et al. (2009). Oxidant Stress in Healthy Normal-weight, Overweight, and Obese Individuals. Obesity. 17: 460–466.

21. Brunelli E, Domanico F, La Russa D et al. (2014). Sex differences in oxidative stress biomarkers. Curr Drug Targets. 15:811-815.

22. Cameron AJ, Boyko EJ, Sicree RA et al. (2008). Central obesity as a precursor to the metabolic syndrome in the Aus Diab study and Mauritius. Obesity, 16(12):2707-16.

23. Carmo JM, da Silva AA, Wang Z et al. (2016). Obesity-induced hypertension: brain signaling pathways. CurrHypertens Rep. 18:58.

24. Casimir GJA and Duchateau J. (2011). Gender differences in inflammatory processes could explain poorer prognosis for males. J Clin Microbiol. 49(1): 478-479.
25. Casimir GJA, Heldenbergh F., Hanssens L. et al. (2010). Gender differences and inflammation: an in vitro model of blood cells stimulation in prepubescent children. Journal of Inflammation. 7:28.
26. Chattopadhyay M, Khemka VK, Chatterjee G et al. (2015). Enhanced ROS production and oxidative damage in subcutaneous white adipose tissue mitochondria in obese and type 2 diabetes subjects. Molecular and Cellular Biochemistry. 399 (1-2):95–103.
27. Cheeseman KH and Slater TF. (1993). An introduction to free radical biochemistry, Br Med Bull. (3):481-93. doi: 10.1093/oxfordjournals.bmb.a072625.
28. Cushman M. (2002). Effects of hormone replacement therapy and estrogen receptor modulators on markers of inflammation and coagulation. Am J Cardiol. 2002; 90: F7-F10
29. Das UN. (2001). Is obesity an inflammatory condition? Nutrition. 17(11-12): 953–966.
30. Di Renzo L, Galvano F, Orlandi1 C et al. (2010). Oxidative Stress in Normal-Weight Obese Syndrome. Obesity. 18 : 2125–2130.
31. Dietz WH, Robinson TN. (2005). Clinical practice. Overweight children and adolescents. N Engl J Med. 352:2100.
32. Dillard CJ and Tappel AL. (1984). Fluorescent damage products of lipid peroxidation. Methods Enzymol. 105: 337-341.
33. Du Clos TW. (2000). Function of C-reactive protein. Ann Med. 32(4):274–8.
34. Eckel N, Li Y, Kuxhaus O, et al. (2018). Transition from metabolic healthy to unhealthy phenotypes and association with cardiovascular disease risk across BMI categories in 90 257 women (the Nurses' Health Study): 30 year follow-up from a prospective cohort study. The lancet Diabetes & endocrinology. 6(9):714–24.
35. Eckel RH, Grundy SM, Zimmet PZ et al. (2005). The Metabolic Syndrome. Lancet, 16-22: 365(9468):1415-28.

36. El-Ansary A, Bjørklund G, Chirumbolo S et al. (2017). Predictive value of selected biomarkers related to metabolism and oxidative stress in children with autism spectrum disorder Metab Brain Dis. 32:1209–1221. DOI 10.1007/s11011-017-0029-x.

37. Elgazar-Carmon V, Rudich A, Hadad N et al. (2008). Neutrophilstransiently infiltrate intra-abdominal fat early in the course of high-fat feeding. Journal of Lipid Research. 49 :1894–1903.

38. Esterbauer H, Lang J, Zadravee S et al. (1984). Detection of malondialdehyde by high performance liquid chromatography. Methods Enzymol. 105: 319-328.

39. Flegal KM, Carroll MD, Ogden CL et al. (2002). Prevalence and trends in obesity among US adults, 1999- 2000," Journal of the American Medical Association. 288 (14): 1723–1727.

40. FlorinelaC˘atoi A, Elena Pârvu A, Andreicut AD et al. (2018). Metabolically Healthy versus Unhealthy Morbidly Obese: Chronic Inflammation, Nitro-Oxidative Stress, and Insulin Resistance. Nutrients. 10: 1199; doi:10.3390/nu10091199.

41. Fortner RT, Tworoger SS, Wu T et al. (2013). Plasma florescent oxidation products and breast cancer risk: repeated measures in the Nurses' Health Study. Breast Cancer Res Treat. 141: 307-316.

42. Foster MW, McMahon TJ, Stamler JS et al. (2003). Nitrosylation in health and disease. 9(4):160-8.

43. Fukui T, Yamauchi K, Maruyama M., et al. (2011). Significance of measuring oxidative stress in lifestyle-related diseases from the viewpoint of correlation between d-ROMs and BAP in Japanese subjects Hypertension Research. 34 : 1041–1045.

44. Furukawa S, Fujita T, Shimabukuro M et al. (2004). Increased oxidative stress in obesity and its impact on metabolic syndrome, J Clinical Investigation. 114 : 1752-1761.

45. Gaita D, Mosteoru S. (2017). Metabolically healthy versus unhealthy obesity and risk for diabetes mellitus and cardiovascular diseases. Cardiovasc Endocrinol. 6(1):23–6.

46. Gallagher D, Visser M, De Meersman RE et al. (1997). Appendicular skeletal muscle mass: effects of age, gender,and ethnicity. J Appl Physiol. 83:229-39.
47. Gao M, Lv J, Yu C, et al. (2020). Metabolically healthy obesity, transition to unhealthy metabolic status, and vascular disease in Chinese adults: A cohort study. PLoS Med. 17(10): e1003351. https://doi.org/10.1371/journal.pmed.
48. Giordano S, Hage FG, Xing D et al. (2015). Estrogen and cardiovascular disease: Is timing everything? The American Journal of the Medical Sciences. 350(1):27-35.
49. Goh LG, Dhaliwal SS, Welborn TA et al. (2014). Anthropometric measurements of general and central obesity and the prediction of cardiovasculardisease risk in women: across-sectional study. BMJ Open. 4:e004138.
50. Goossens G H. (2017). The Metabolic Phenotype in Obesity: Fat Mass, Body Fat Distribution, and Adipose Tissue Function. Obese Facts. 10:207-215.
51. Government of India. (2016). Ministry of Statistics & Programme Implementation. Elderly in India.
52. Gray DS. (1989). Diagnosis and prevalence of obesity. Med Clin North Am. 73:1-13.
53. Grundy SM, Barnett JP. (1990). Metabolic and health complications of obesity. Dis Mon. 36:641–731.
54. Hackam DG, Redelmeier DA. (2006). JAMA. 11;296(14):1731-2.
55. Halliwell B. (1989). Free radicals, reactive oxygen species and human disease: a critical evaluation with special reference to atherosclerosis, Exp Pathol. 70(6): 737–757.
56. Han Y, Kim M, JinYoo H et al. (2019). Metabolically Unhealthy Overweight Individuals Have High Lysophosphatide Levels, Phospholipase Activity, and Oxidative Stress. Diabetes. 68, 320-lb(Supplement 1).
57. Hackam DG, Redelmeier DA. (2006). JAMA. 11;296(14):1731-2.
58. Halliwell B. (1989). Free radicals, reactive oxygen species and human disease: a critical evaluation with special reference to atherosclerosis, Exp Pathol. 70(6): 737–757.
59. Han Y, Kim M, JinYoo H et al. (2019). Metabolically Unhealthy Overweight

Individuals Have High Lysophosphatide Levels, Phospholipase Activity, and Oxidative Stress. Diabetes. 68, 320-lb(Supplement 1).

60. Harman D. (1992). Free radical theory of aging, Mutation Research. 275(3-6):257-66.

61. Hashimoto Y, Hamaguchi M, Tanaka M et al. (2018). Metabolically healthy obesity without fatty liver and risk of incident type 2 diabetes: A meta-analysis of prospective cohort studies. Obesity Research & Clinical Practice. 12 (1) : 4-15.

62. Haslam, D. (2007). Obesity: a medical history. Obes. Rev. 8: 31-36.

63. Hermsdorff HH, Zulet MA, Bressan J. et al. (2008). Effect of diet on the low-grade and chronic inflammation associated with obesity and metabolic syndrome. Endocrinol Nutr. 55: 409–19.

64. Iacobini C, Pugliese G, Fantauzzi FC et al. (2019). Metabolically healthy versus metabolically unhealthy obesity. Metabolism Clinical and Experimental. 92, 51-60.

65. Jensen MK, Wang Y, Rimm EB et al. (2013). Fluorescent oxidation products and risk of coronary heart disease: a prospective study in women. J Am Heart Assoc. 2: e000195.

66. Jung CH, Lee WJ, Song KH. (2017). Metabolically healthy obesity: a friend or foe? Korean J Intern Med.;32:611–21.

67. Kanter R. (2012). Global Gender Disparities in Obesity: A Review, Rebecca Kanter2,3 and Benjamin Caballero2 ã2012 American Society for Nutrition. Adv. Nutr. 3: 491–498.

68. Karalis KP, Giannogonas P, Kodela E. et al. (2009). Mechanisms of obesity and related pathology: linking immune responses to metabolic stress. FEBS J 276:5747–5754.

69. Karelis AD, Rabasa-Lhoret R. (2008) Inclusion of C-reactive protein in the identification of metabolically healthy but obese (MHO) individuals. Diabetes Metab. 34 (2):183–4.

70. Kelli HM, Corrigan FE, Heinl RE et al. (2017). Relation of Changes in Body Fat Distribution to Oxidative Stress. Am J Cardiol. 120 (12):2289-2293.

71. Khawaja KI, Mian SA, Fatima A et al. (2018). Phenotypic and metabolic

dichotomy in obesity: clinical, biochemical and immunological correlates of metabolically divergent obese phenotypes in healthy South Asian adults. Singapore Med J. 59(8): 431-438.

72. Kim IY, Han KD, Kim DH et al. (2019). Women with Metabolic Syndrome and General Obesity Are at a Higher Risk for Significant Hyperuricemia Compared to Men. J Clin Med 8(6):837. doi: 10.3390/ jcm8060837.

73. Kintscher U, Hartge M, Hess K et al. (2008). T-lymphocyte infiltration in visceral adipose tissue: a primary event in adipose tissue inflammation and the development of obesity mediated insulin resistance. Arterioscler Thromb Vasc Biol. 28:1304–1310.

74. Korotkova EI, Bashkim M, Elena VD et al. (2011). Study of OH• Radicals in Human Serum Blood of HealthyIndividuals and Those with Pathological SchizophreniaInt. J. Mol. Sci.;12, 401-409.

75. Kowalska K. and Milnerowicz H. (2016). The Influence of Age and Gender on the Pro/Antioxidant Status in Young Healthy People, Annals of Clinical & Laboratory Science. 46 : 5.

76. Kramer CK, Zinman B, Retnakaran R. (2013). Are metabolically healthy overweight and obesity benign conditions?: A systematic review and meta-analysis. Ann Intern Med. 159(11): 758–69.

77. Laaksonen DE., Niskanen L, Nyyssönen K et al. (2004). C-reactive protein and the development of the metabolic syndrome and diabetes in middle-aged men. 47(8):1403-10.

78. Leal V de O and Mafra D. (2013). Adipokines in obesity. Clin Chim Acta. 419:87–94.

79. Lee J. Adipose tissue macrophages in the development of obesity induced inflammation, insulin resistance and type 2 Diabetes. Arch Pharm Res. 2013;36:208–22.

80. Lee JJ, Freeland-Graves JH, Pepper M R et al. (2014). Predictive Equations for Central Obesity via Anthropometrics, Stereovision Imaging and MRI in Adults. Obesity. 22, 852–862.

81. Lee MJ, Wu Y, Fried SK. (2010). Adipose tissue remodeling in Pathophysiology of obesity. Curr Opin Clin NutrMetab Care. 13:371–6.

82. Lejawa, M., Osadnik, K., Osadnik, T et al. (2021). Association of Metabolically Healthy and Unhealthy Obesity Phenotypes with Oxidative Stress Parameters and Telomere Length in Healthy Young Adult Men. Analysis of MAGNETIC study. Antioxidants 10,93.

83. Levine LR., Garland D, Oliver NC. et al. (1990). Determination of carbonyl content in oxidatively modified proteins, Methods in Enzymology.186:464-478.

84. Li X, Fang P, Mai J et al. (2013). Targeting mitochondrial reactive oxygen species as novel therapy for inflammatory diseases and cancers. J Hematol Oncol. 6:19.

85. Marie C. (2005). Sex differences in cardiovascular disease and hypertension: involvement of the renin-angiotensin system, Hypertension, 46(3):475–476.

86. Marklund S and Marklund G. (1974) Involovement of the superoxide anion radical in the autooxidation of pyrogallol and a convenient assay for superoxide dismutase.European Journal of Biochem;16-47(3):469-74.

87. Malik VS, Willett WC, Hu FB. (2013). Global obesity: trends, risk factors and policy implications. Nature Reviews Endocrinology. 9 (1): 13–27.

88. Marrocco I, Altieri F, Peluso I et al. (2017). Measurement and clinical significance of biomarkers of oxidative stress in humans. Oxidative Medicine and Cellular Longevity.:32.

89. Maury E, Brichard SM. (2010). Adipokine dysregulation, adipose tissue inflammation and metabolic syndrome. Mol Cell Endocrinol. 15;314(1):1-16.

90. McLaughlin T, Lamendola C, Liu A et al. (2011). Preferential fat deposition in subcutaneous versus visceral depots is associated with insulin sensitivity. Journal of Clinical Endocrinology and Metabolism. 96 (11):1756–60.

91. Medhi GK, Mahanta J. (2007). Population ageing in India: health promotion through life course approach. CurrSci. 93:1046.

92. Messier V, Karelis AD, Robillard ME et al. (2011). Metabolically healthy but obese individuals: relationship with hepatic enzymes. Metabolism; 35(7):971-81.

93. Meigs JB, Lipinska I, Kathiresan S et al. (2007). Visceral and subcutaneous adipose tissue volumes are cross-sectionally related to markers of

inflammation and oxidative stress. The Framingham Heart Study. Circulation. 116:11:1234–1241.

94. Milewicz A, Jedrzejuk D, Dunajska K et al. (2010). Waist circumference and serum adiponectin levels in obese and non-obese postmenopausal women. 65, 3, 272 – 275.

95. Misra A. (2015). Ethnic-Specific Criteria for Classification of Body Mass Index: A Perspective for Asian Indians and American Diabetes Association Position Statement. Diabetes technology & therapeutics; 17: (9) 667-71.

96. Mittal PC and Ruchi Kant. (2009). Correlation of increased oxidative stress to body weight in disease-free post menopausal women. Clinical Biochemistry. 42:1007–1011.

97. Muller A and Sies H. (1984). Assay of ethane and pentane from isolated organs and cells. In: Methods Enzymol. Pcker L (Eds.) Vol 105, Academic Press, New York, 311-319.

98. Mundy AL, Haas E, Bhattacharya I et al., 2007 Endothelin stimulates vascular hydroxyl radical formation: effect of obesityAm J PhysiolRegulIntegr Comp Physiol 2007; 293: R2218–R2224

99. National Cholesterol Education Program (NCEP). (2010). Expert Panel on Detection E, and Treatment of High Blood Cholesterol in Adults (Adult Treatment Panel III). Third Report of the National Cholesterol Education Program (NCEP) Expert Panel on Detection, Evaluation, and Treatment of High Blood Cholesterol in Adults (Adult Treatment Panel III) Final Report. Circulation. 106:3143-3421.

100. NHLBI Expert Panel. (2002). author. Clinical guidelines on the identification, evaluation, and treatment of overweight and obesity in adults: evidence report. Bethesda, MD: NIH; NIH publication no. 02-4084.

101. Niehaus W G, Samuelsson B. (1968). Formation of Malonaldehyde from Phospholipid Arachidonate during Microsomal Lipid Peroxidation. European Journal of Biochemistry Banner. 1432-1033.

102. Nijhawan LP, Janodia MD, Muddukrishna BS. et al. (2013). Informed consent: Issues and challenges. J Adv Pharm Technol Res. 4 (3):134–140.

103. Nishimura S, Manabe I, Nagasaki M et al. (2009). CD8+ effector T cells

contribute to macrophage recruitment and adipose tissue inflammation in obesity. Nature Medicine 15 914–920.

104. Ogden CL, Carroll MD, Curtin LR, et al. (2006). Prevalence of overweight and obesity in the United States, 1999–2004. JAMA (2006) 295:1549–55.

105. Onat A, Karadeniz Y, Tusun E et al. (2016). Advances in understanding gender difference in cardiometabolic disease risk. Expert Rev Cardiovasc Ther. 14(4):513–23.

106. Ozata M, Mergen M, Oktenli C et al. (2002). Increased oxidative stress and hypozincemia in male obesity. Clin Biochem, 35(8):627–31.

107. Pajunen P, Kotronen A, Korpi-HyovaltiE,et al. (2011). Metabolically healthy and unhealthy obesity phenotypes in the general population: the FIN-D2D Survey. BMC Public Health;11:754.

108. Pasquali R, Casimirri LF, Labate AMM, et al. (1995). Body weight, fat distribution and the menopausal status in women. Maturitas. 21(3):259 (1).

109. Pihl E, Zilmer K, Kullisaar T. (2006). Atherogenic inflammatory and oxidative stress markers in relation to overweight values in male former athletes. *Int. J. Obesity. 30*, 141–146.

110. Pinnick KE, Nicholson G, Manolopoulos KN et al. (2014). Distinct developmental profile of lower-body adipose tissue defines resistance against obesity-associated metabolic complications. Diabetes. 63: 3785–379.

111. Pi-Sunyer FX. (2006). The relation of adipose tissue to cardiometabolic risk. Clin Cornerstone.8(4):14–23.

112. Pi-Sunyer FX. (1999). Obesity. In editors. Modern Nutrition in Health and Disease. Williams and Wilkins Baltimore. 1395–418.7.

113. Power ML, Schulkin J. (2008). Sex differences in fat storage, fat metabolism, and the health risks from obesity: possible evolutionary origins. Br J Nutr. 99:931–40.

114. Pradhan AD, Manson JE, Rifai N et al. (2001). C-reactive protein, interleukin 6, and risk of developing type 2 diabetes mellitus. J Am Med Assoc. 286(3):327–34.

115. Primeau V, Coderre L, Karelis AD et al. (2011). Characterizing the profile of obese patients who are metabolically healthy. Int J Obes (Lond); 35: 971–981.

116. Purty AJ, Bazroy J, Kar M et al. (2006). Morbidity pattern among the elderly population in the rural area of Tamil Nadu, India. Turkey J Med Sci. 36:45-50.
117. Phillips CM. (2013). Metabolically healthy obesity: definitions, determinants and clinical implications. Rev Endocr Metab Disord. 14(3): 219–27.
118. Reuser M, Bonneux L, Willekens F. (2008). The burden of mortality of obesity at middle and old age is small. A life table analysis of the US Health and Retirement Survey. Eur J Epidemiol. 23(9):601-607.
119. Rexknagel RO and Glende EA. (1984). Spectrophotometric detection of lipid conjugated dienes, Methods Enzymol 1984;105:331-7.
120. Roberts CK, Sindhu KK. (2009). Oxidative stress and metabolic syndrome. Life Sci 84:705–712.
121. Rotruck JT, Pope AL, Ganther HE et al. (1973). Selenium: biochemical role as a component of glutathione peroxidase.Science. 179(4073):588-90.
122. Ruiz-Larrea MB, Martin C, Martinez R, et al. (2000). Antioxidant activities of estrogens against aqueous and lipophillic radicals; differences between phenol and catechol estrogens. Chem Phys Lipids. 105:179–88.
123. Rush EC, Goedecke JH, Jennings C et al. (2007). BMI, fat and muscle differences in urban women of five ethnicities from two countries. Int J Obes (Lond); 31: 1232–1239.
124. Sánchez AF, Santillán EM, Bautista M et al. (2011). Inflammation, Oxidative Stress, and Obesity. Int. J. Mol. Sci. 12, 3117-3132.
125. Schillaci G, Pasqualini L, Vaudo G. (2003). Effect of body weight changes on 24-hour blood pressure and left ventricular mass; a 4-year follow-up. Am J Hypertens. 16:634–9.
126. Schmidt MI, Duncan BB, Sharrett AR et al. (1999). Markers of inflammation and prediction of diabetes mellitus in adults (Atherosclerosis Risk in Communities study): a cohort study. Lancet. 353:1649–52.
127. Shaharyar S, Roberson LL, Jamal O. (2015). Obesity and Metabolic Phenotypes (Metabolically Healthy and Unhealthy Variants) Are Significantly Associated with Prevalence of Elevated C-Reactive Protein and Hepatic Steatosis in a Large Healthy Brazilian Population Journal of Obesity Volume 2015, Article ID 178526, 6.

128. Shoelson SE, Lee J, Goldfine Ab et al. (2006). Inflammation and insulin resistance. J Clin Invest. 116: 1793-801.
129. Sies H, Stahl W, Sevanian A. (2005). Nuritional, dietary and post prandial oxidative stress. J. Nutr. 135: 969-972.
130. Sims EAH. (1982). Characterization of the syndromes of obesity. In Textbook of Diabetes mellitus and obesity. Williams and Wilkins. 219–226.
131. Singh S, Dwivedi A, Kumar S et al. (2019). Total Antioxidant Status and Other Markers to Distinguish Severely Obese Volunteers with and without Metabolic Syndrome. Food and Nutrition Sciences; 10, 648-663.
132. Sinha AK. (1974). Colorimetric assay of catalase. Anal Biochem.. 47(2):389-94.
133. Slater TF. (1983). Lipid peroxidation.Biochem. Soc. Trans. 10:70-71.
134. Slater TF. (1984). Free radical mechanisms in tissue injury. Biochem. 222: 1-15.
135. Spiegelman BM and Flier JS. (1996). Adipogenesis and obesity: rounding out the big picture. Cell. 87: 377–389.
136. Stadtman,ER. (2004). Role of oxidant species in ageing. Sci. Curr. Med. Chem. 11: 1105-1112.
137. Stadtman,ER. (2001). Protein oxidation in age related diseases. Ann. New York Acad. Sci. 928: 22-38.
138. Stefan H, Haring HU, Hu FB et al. (2013). Metabolically healthy obesity: epidemiology, mechanisms, and clinical implications. The Lancet Diabetes & Endocrinology. 1(2):152-62.
139. Sun K, Kusminski CM, Scherer PE. (2011). Adipose tissue remodeling and obesity. J Clin Investig. 121:2094–101.
140. Tchkonia T, Thomou T, Zhu Y et al. (2013). Mechanisms and metabolic implications of regional differences among fat depots. Cell Metabolism. 17: 644–656.
141. Thomas T, Ruth B, Konard J. (2001). Surveillance of stroke: a global perspective. Int J Epidemiol. 30(Suppl. 1):S11-6.
142. Tzanetakou IP, Katsilambros NL, Benetos A et al. (2012). Is obesity linked to aging?: adipose tissue and the role of telomeres. Ageing Res Rev. 11, 220–

229.

143. Tian S, Liu Y, Feng Ao, et al. (2020). Sex-Specific Differences in the Association of Metabolically Healthy Obesity with Hyperuricemia and a Network Perspective in Analyzing Factors Related to Hyperuricemia Front. Endocrinol. 11:573452.

144. Tianying W, Rifai NL. Roberts II LJ et al. (2004). Stability of Measurements of Biomarkers ofOxidative Stress in Blood Over 36 Hours. Cancer Epidemiol Biomarkers Prev.13(8).

145. Singh S and Mittal PC. (2019). Title of thesis, Biochemical Correlates of the Metabolic Syndrome.

146. Turrens JF, Freeman BA, Levitt JG. et al. (1982). The effect of hypoxia on superoxide production in lung submitochondrial particles. Biochem. Biophys. Acta. 217: 401-410.

147. Valentine RJ, McAuley E, Vieira VJ et al. (2009). Sex differences in the relationship between obesity, C-reactive protein, physical activity, depression, sleep quality and fatigue in older adults. Brain Behav Immun. 23: 643-648.

148. Van Vliet-Ostaptchouk JV, Nuotio ML, Slagter SN, Doiron D, Fischer K, Foco L, [6]et al. The prevalence of metabolic syndrome and metabolically healthy obesity in Europe: a collaborative analysis of ten large cohort studies. BMC Endocrine Disorders. 2014;14(1):9

149. Vehapoglu A, Turkmen S, Goknar N et al. (2016). Reduced antioxidant capacity and increased subclinical inflammation markers in prepubescent obese children and their relationship with nutritional markers and metabolic parameters, Redox Report. 21:6,271-280.

150. Venturini D, Simão AN, Scripes NA et al. (2012). Evaluation of oxidative stress in overweight subjects with or without metabolic syndrome. Obesity. 20:2361–6.

151. Villareal DT, Apovian CM, Kushner RF et al. (2005). Obesity in older adults: technical review and position statement of the American Society for Nutrition and NAASO, The Obesity Society. Obes Res. 13 : 1849–1863.

152. Vincent HK, Innes KE, Vincent KR. (2007). Oxidative stress and potential interventions to reduce oxidative stress in overweight and obesity. Diabetes,

Obesity and Metabolism. 9: 813–839.

153. Wagner G, Lindroos-Christensen J, Einwallner E et al. (2017). HO-1 inhibits preadipocyte proliferation and differentiation at the onset of obesity via ROS dependent activation of Akt2. Scientific Reports. 7: 40881.

154. Weiss R, Dziura J, Burgert TS et al. (2004). Obesity and the metabolic syndrome in children and adolescents. N Engl J Med. 350:2362-2374.

155. Wellen KE and Hotamisligil GS. (2005). Inflammation, stress, and diabetes. Journal of Clinical Investigation. 115 (5): 1111–1119.

156. WHO (1995). Physical Status: The Use and Interpretation of Anthropometry. WHO Technical Report Series No. 854, World Health Organization, Geneva.

157. WHO (2011). Global Health and Aging, National Institute on Aging National Institutes of Health U.S. Department of Health and Human Services.

158. WHO Expert Consultation (2000). Appropriate body-mass index for Asian populations and its implications for policy and intervention strategies. Lancet. 363(9403):157-63.

159. WHO (2000). Obesity: preventing and managing the global epidemic. WHO Technical Report Series number 894, Geneva.

160. WHO (1995). Physical Status: The Use and Interpretation of Anthropometry. WHO Technical Report Series No. 854, World Health Organization, Geneva.

161. WHO (2008). Waist circumference and waist-hip ratio: Report of a WHO expert consultation, Geneva.

162. Wiklund P, Pekkala S, Autio R et al. (2014). Serum metabolic profiles in overweight and obese women with and without metabolic syndrome. Diabetology & Metabolic Syndrome. 6,40

163. Wildman RP, Muntner P, Reynolds K et al. (2008). The obese without cardiometabolic risk factor clustering and the normal weight with cardiometabolic risk factor clustering: prevalence and correlates of 2 phenotypes among the US population (NHANES 1999–2004)," Archives of Internal Medicine. 168 (15):1617–1624.

164. Wing RR, Matthews KA, Kuller LH et al. (1991). Weight gain at the time of menopause. Arch Intern Med. 151(1):97–102.

165. Wisdom SJ, Wilson R, McKillop JH et al. (1991). Antioxidant systems in

normal pregnancy and in pregnancy-induced hypertension. Am J Obstet Gynecol. 165:170–74.

166. World Population Ageing. (2019). Highlights, Department of Economic and Social Affairs Population Division, United Nations.

167. Wu T, Rifai N, Willett WC et al. (2007). Plasma fluorescent oxidation products: independent predictors of coronary heart disease in men. Am J Epidemiol. 166: 544-551.

168. Xu, H, Barnes, GT, Yang, Q et al. (2003). Chronic inflammation in fat plays a crucial role in the development of obesity-related insulin resistance. J. Clin. Investig. 112:1821–1830.

169. Yagi K. (1997). Female hormones act as natural antioxidants—a survey of our research. Acta Biochim Pol. 44:701–9.

170. Yoshida Y, Umeno A, Shichiri M et al. (2013). Lipid peroxidation biomarkers for evaluating oxidative stress and assessing antioxidant capacity in vivo. J Clin Biochem Nutr. 52:9-16.

171. Zelko IN, Mariani TJ, Folz RJ. (2002). Superoxide dismutase multigene family: a comparison of the CuZn-SOD (SOD1), Mn-SOD (SOD2), and EC-SOD (SOD3) gene structures, evolution, and expression. Free Radical Biology and Medicine. 33(3):337-349.

CPSIA information can be obtained
at www.ICGtesting.com
Printed in the USA
LVHW040615201222
735554LV00012B/527